MW01097154

The **best** friends™
Approach to
Dementia Care

Praise for this edition of
The Best Friends Approach to Dementia Care

"The Best Friends™ philosophy has changed the face of dementia over the last two decades. . . . This new edition will teach you everything you thought you already knew."
—**Amelia Schafer, M.S.**, Vice President of Programs, Alzheimer's Association, Colorado Chapter

"Whether your program serves six persons with dementia or six hundred, this new edition will become an invaluable resource. In addition to its practical tips for quality dementia care, the book offers insights into how you can obtain staff buy-in, implement your ideas, and sustain a great program over time."
—**Tom Cullen**, CEO & Owner, Community Care Options

"The Best Friends philosophy, rich in relationships and engagement, and respectful of human rights, provides a lasting foundation for dementia friendly communities and quality care."
—**Marc Wortmann**, Executive Director, Alzheimer's Disease International

"This book should be 'must reading' for care partners, both professional and family. It is practical, offering clear ways to implement all aspects of this extraordinary program. Living with memory loss can be a very frightening journey, but when surrounded by Best Friends who help you continue to engage in life, the journey can still have many moments of joy."
—**Joyce Simard, M.S.W.**, Geriatric Consultant, Associate Professor, Western Sydney University, and author, *The End-of-Life Namaste Care™ Program for People with Dementia*

"I strongly recommend this book as an essential resource for anyone and everyone working in a care setting."
—**Padma Genesh, B.Sc.**, MBBS, B.A., Learning Specialist, Learning and Support Services, Alzheimer Society of Calgary, Canada

"Two decades ago, Bell and Troxel's Best Friends™ approach affirmed the primary importance of relationship in supporting well-being for people living with dementia. It is great to see this thoughtful update of a classic and time-honored model for engagement and care."
—**G. Allen Power, M.D., FACP**, author of *Dementia Beyond Drugs* and *Dementia Beyond Disease*

"The Best Friends books have become our go-to resource for ideas and inspirations about quality dementia care. This new edition raises the bar as it challenges us to develop authentic relationships and meaningful activities and to create outstanding programs."
—**Dina Newsom**, Expressions™ Product Manager, Prestige Senior Living, Vancouver, WA

"Best Friends is helping to establish ourselves as a center of excellence in dementia care throughout our region."
—**Dan Lavender**, President & CEO, Moorings Park, Naples, FL

"We embrace the Best Friends philosophy in all our Life Guidance® memory care neighborhoods across the United States. This new edition of the classic Best Friends book is full of contemporary best practices and practical tips for successfully navigating the challenges of dementia care. It will be a valuable resource for our staff as we encourage relationships and meaningful activities to create a successful day."
—**Tom Alaimo**, Vice President, Memory Care Operations (Life Guidance®), Atria Senior Living, Louisville, KY

"[The Best Friends approach has] changed the history of dementia care in our country since Best Friends is now included in the developing Dementia Strategy of Hungary!"
—**Zsuzsa Kovacsics, M.S.W.**, Administrator, Máriaremete Nursing Home, Budapest, Hungary

"The Best Friends philosophy is perfect for home care settings and beautifully supports the Home Instead Senior Care® network's To Us, It's Personal® philosophy. The person with dementia benefits from this loving approach and our network's professional CAREgivers℠ can manage the challenges of dementia with wisdom and creativity."
—**Jeff Huber**, President & CEO, Home Instead, Inc.

"Bell and Troxel, in their inspiring book, . . . have shown me the way home and given me new confidence that I am not alone, that I don't have to fight Alzheimer's myself. . . . [They] are partners who can lead."
—**Greg O'Brien**, author, On Pluto: Inside the Mind of Alzheimer's

"The Best Friends approach really works, attracting volunteers and building a fantastic day of activities and engagement. Our day center participants . . . have felt known, loved, and valued, as have I."
—**Linda Rector**, volunteer, Best Friends™ Day Center, Lexington, KY

Additional titles available on Best Friends™ care practices

The Best Friends Book of Alzheimer's Activities
Volume One
Volume Two
by Virginia Bell, David Troxel, Tonya Cox & Robin Hamon

The Best Friends Staff:
Building a Culture of Care in Alzheimer's Programs
by Virginia Bell & David Troxel

The Best Friends Daily Planner
by Virginia Bell & David Troxel

Los Mejores Amigos en el Cuidado de Alzheimer
by Virginia Bell & David Troxel

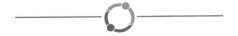

To order, contact Health Professions Press, Inc.
Post Office Box 10624 • Baltimore, MD 21285-0624
1-888-337-8808
www.healthpropress.com

For questions about quantity discounts or training,
including training for Best Friends™ Master Trainer Certification,
contact bestfriends@healthpropress.com

www.facebook.com/bestfriendsapproach
@HealthProPress

The **best** friends™ Approach to Dementia Care

SECOND EDITION

by

Virginia Bell, M.S.W.
David Troxel, M.P.H.

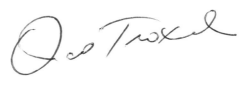

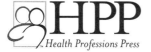

Baltimore • London • Sydney

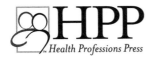

Health Professions Press, Inc.
Post Office Box 10624
Baltimore, Maryland 21285-0624

www.healthpropress.com

Interior design by Mindy Dunn.
Cover design by Erin Geoghegan.

Typeset by Absolute Service, Inc., Towson, Maryland.
Manufactured in the United States of America by Maple Press, York, Pennsylvania.

Best Friends™ and the (**best** friends˜ logo are trademarks of Health Professions Press, Inc.

Library of Congress Cataloging-in-Publication Data

Names: Bell, Virginia, author. | Troxel, David, author.
Title: The best friends approach to dementia care / by Virginia Bell, David Troxel.
Other titles: The best friends approach to Alzheimer's care
Description: Second edition. | Baltimore, Maryland : Health Professions Press, Inc., [2017] | Preceded by The best friends approach to Alzheimer's care / Virginia Bell and David Troxel. c1997. | Includes bibliographical references and index.
Identifiers: LCCN 2016029960 (print) | LCCN 2016031057 (ebook) | ISBN 9781932529968 (pbk.) | ISBN 9781938870637 (epub)
Subjects: | MESH: Dementia | Interpersonal Relations | Long-Term Care--methods
Classification: LCC RC523 (print) | LCC RC523 (ebook) | NLM WT 155 | DDC 362.1968/31--dc23
LC record available at https://lccn.loc.gov/2016029960

British Library Cataloguing-in-Publication data are available from the British Library.

Contents

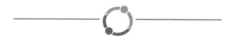

About the Authors

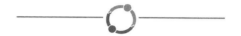

Virginia Bell and David Troxel are recognized internationally for their groundbreaking and innovative work helping people with dementia, their families, and professional care partners. With decades of experience working in university, community, and adult day center settings, they have pioneered the development of an effective, meaningful model of dementia care in the Best Friends™ philosophy.

Virginia Bell, M.S.W., is a pioneer in the field, having founded one of the first dementia-specific adult day programs, the award-winning Helping Hand Adult Day Center (funded in part through the prestigious Robert Wood Johnson Foundation). Since opening its doors in 1984, it has served as a model for many other programs nationally. After being renamed the Best Friends™ Adult Day Center, it also became a "teaching-learning center" for social work, nursing, and medical students from the University of Kentucky.

Bell earned her master's in social work from the University of Kentucky, where she also counseled families at the university's Sanders-Brown Center on Aging and learned to appreciate the unique challenges faced by people with dementia and their care partners. Since then, she has published numerous journal articles and book chapters and has co-authored six books about the Best Friends™ approach with David Troxel.

She has been recognized at the regional, state, and national levels for her leadership and good works, including prestigious awards from the American Society on Aging, the University and the state of Kentucky, and the national Alzheimer's Association, and she has served on two Governor's task forces on aging and Alzheimer's disease. Bell has been a Program Consultant for the Greater Kentucky/Southern Indiana Chapter of the Alzheimer's Association and has lectured in more than

30 countries, including presentations for 26 Alzheimer's Disease International conferences.

David Troxel, M.P.H., is a consultant about dementia across the continuum of aging care. He served for a decade as president and CEO of the California Central Coast Alzheimer's Association, Santa Barbara, California (1994–2004), and has been a member of the Ethics Advisory Panel for the national Alzheimer's Association.

After earning his master's in public health from Rutgers University, Troxel worked at the University of Kentucky Sanders-Brown Center on Aging, which at the time was one of only ten federally funded Alzheimer's research centers in the country. It was there he met and began to collaborate with Virginia Bell to improve education and services in the state of Kentucky for people with dementia and their care partners. He was the first executive director of the Lexington/Bluegrass chapter of the Alzheimer's Association (now called the Greater Kentucky and Southern Indiana chapter) and, together with Virginia Bell, he won an unprecedented four Excellence in Program Awards from the national Alzheimer's Association for his chapter's patient and family programs.

Troxel has also been a family care partner, supporting his mother, Dorothy, who passed away from Alzheimer's disease in 2008 after a 10-year journey with the disease.

Troxel is a popular speaker for regional and national events and is known worldwide for his writing and teaching in the fields of Alzheimer's and long-term care. In addition to the books he has co-written with Virginia Bell on their Best Friends™ philosophy, together they have written a series of influential journal articles on topics ranging from spirituality, to staff training and development, to person-centered care, including the widely reprinted Best Friends™ Dementia Bill of Rights.

**To learn more about Virginia's and David's work,
visit them on the Web:**
www.bestfriendsapproach.com
http://bestfriends.healthpropress.com
www.facebook.com/bestfriendsapproach

Acknowledgments

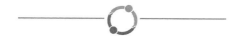

We have many people to thank who have stood by us since we began our work in dementia care.

Our friends and colleagues at the University of Kentucky Sanders-Brown Center on Aging deserve special acknowledgment. The late Dr. David Wekstein brought us together as colleagues at the center; we thank its talented staff and alumni, who include Dr. Deborah Danner, Dr. Linda Kuder, and Marie Smart. Robin Hamon continues her work at the center and is a co-author of our activity books. The late Dr. William Markesbery was particularly generous in his support.

Tonya Cox of Christian Care Communities has been a longtime friend, colleague, and co-author and she contributed her wisdom from years of experience in the field to Part 3 of this book.

We thank past and present staff and volunteers at the Best Friends Day Center in Lexington, Kentucky, for their ongoing commitment to this model program. This award-winning adult day center was the birthplace of the Best Friends™ approach and remains an influential source of learning and inspiration.

Two chapters of the Alzheimer's Association have provided a home and support for our work. The Greater Kentucky and Southern Indiana Chapter of the Alzheimer's Association (based in Louisville) and the Central Coast Chapter of the Alzheimer's Association (based in Santa Barbara) supported Virginia's and David's work. A special thank you to Kentucky volunteers and staff, including Claire Macfarlane, Marie Masters, Jane Owen, Margaret Patterson, Linda and Ray Rector, and Jan Cerel. A special thank you to Santa Barbara volunteers and staff, past and present, including Barbara Rose, Charlie Zimmer, Lol Sorensen, the late Elayne Brill, the late Dr. Erno Daniel, Dr. Robert Harbaugh, Debbie McConnell, Cynthia Thompson, and Julian Dean.

Other notable supporters and friends include Tom Alaimo, Nancy Schier Anzelmo, Molly Carpenter, Dr. Steven DeKosky, Dr. Elizabeth Edgerly, Hollie Fowler, Dr. Nori Graham, Berna Huebner, Dr. Linda Hewett, Kay Kallander, Dan Kuhn, Celeste Lynch, Cynthia Lilly, Dina Newsom, Dr. Al Power, Joanne Rader, Dr. Peter Reed, and Mark Steele—all of whom have contributed greatly to quality of life for many persons with dementia and their care partners.

A number of long-term care companies and organizations have contributed to this book. Special thanks to our Best Friends at American Baptist Homes of the West (ABHOW), Americare Senior Living, Atria Senior Living, Christian Care Communities, Elmcroft Senior Living, Heritage Community of Kalamazoo (Michigan), Home Instead Senior Care, Moorings Park, Prestige Care, The Plaza Assisted Living (Hawaii), and Touchmark Senior Living.

We thank the growing group of Best Friends Master Trainers who are taking our work and message to family and professional care settings in the United States and Canada. The work and ideas of some of these Master Trainers are cited in this edition.

The Robert Wood Johnson Foundation supported our work with an early grant to the Best Friends Day Center.

The Steele-Reese Foundation supported our early work and education about caregiving issues in rural communities.

Dr. William Stivelman and the Mary Oakley Foundation remain strong supporters of our work, including our Spanish-language edition and outreach.

We wish to acknowledge Dr. Nori Graham, Marc Wortmann, and our friends at Alzheimer's Disease International for their work to support care partners around the world.

Kathy Laurenhue is a long-time friend and colleague whose creative writings in the United States and internationally have changed the face of dementia care. Kathy contributed to thinking on engagement and volunteerism included in this book.

Anne Basye runs our Best Friends website and social media and deserves special mention as a close collaborator who reviewed, edited, and shepherded the book manuscript to completion.

Matt Ehrmann contributed design and content ideas and M. Skrzynski is the talented artist who created the new "comic book art" featured in this book.

Our friends and colleagues at Health Professions Press, including Melissa Behm, Mary Magnus, Lisa Minick, and Julie Chávez, support us with an ongoing partnership and sharp editorial eye.

Finally, a few personal acknowledgments.

From Virginia Bell: To the staff that I have met all over the world who exemplify the Best Friends approach, and to my husband Wayne Bell.

From David Troxel: To my late parents Fred and Dorothy Troxel, and to my partner Ron Spingarn.

Preface

Our Best Friends Journey

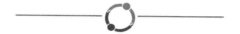

When we first conceived of the Best Friends™ approach, public awareness of the challenges of Alzheimer's disease and other dementias was low. For most of the 20th century, during what Virginia Bell calls the "winter" of Alzheimer's disease, people with dementia were thought to be belligerent, crazy, and even dangerous. Everyone with dementia was treated the same way; all too often, they were wrenched from their loved ones because confinement was sometimes considered the only solution. It wasn't uncommon for people with dementia to be committed to an institution with no attention to basic rights.

In the 1980s, when we worked at the University of Kentucky Alzheimer's Disease Research Center, the landscape was still a difficult one for family and professional care partners:

- There was little public awareness of Alzheimer's disease and other dementias.
- Few services and support programs were available.
- Physicians were largely uninformed about dementia.
- Professional care staff had little training in dementia care.
- Specialized memory care neighborhoods and programs were in their infancy.
- The "treatment" for dementia was still conservative, focusing on safety and routine rather than enrichment and quality of life.

As a result, families and care partners felt (and often were) all alone as they faced tremendous difficulties providing care for the person with dementia. How should one respond to repetitive questions or accusations, cope with aggression, address exit seeking, or respond to other challenges? Was there any way to enhance the quality of life of the person with dementia? How could family members cope with their own physical, emotional, and financial stress? How could care staff succeed? Back then, we didn't have many answers.

Frustrated by the lack of services and creativity in care, Virginia started one of the first adult day centers in the country for persons with Alzheimer's disease or other dementias. Many centers viewed their purpose primarily as a respite program to give families a welcome break. Virginia believed the centers could be much more. The Best Friends Day Center, which opened in 1984 with staff support from the University of Kentucky and a group of caring volunteers, set out to offer a loving, caring place packed with meaningful relationships, music, dance, good food, and activity.

Initially there was concern that Virginia and her team might have gotten in over their heads. Several prominent professionals were skeptical that the center could succeed. One national expert even predicted that violent behavior would be the norm. Families were also concerned: Would their loved one be disruptive or have an unhappy experience while at the day center?

Instead, something began happening that could only be described as magical, as participants were treated with respect and affection. Jane Owen, one of the original volunteers, confirms this:

> The families would bring their loved ones, and you could sometimes see them arguing and fighting as they came in. We weren't really sure what would work but decided to create a party atmosphere. This seemed to capture the participants' attention. It was like they were with company and consequently they were on their best behavior. Virginia called it a therapeutic environment, but I just called it fun and friendship.

Why did someone with dementia, who was so difficult for his or her family member, do so well with the staff at the center? The answer was simple. Through programming and staff, Virginia was creating a "therapeutic environment." Simply defined, a therapeutic, healing environment draws on knowledge of the history, preferences, and pastimes of the person with dementia; involves communicating with the person in ways that affirm and respect; and offers activities, planned and spontaneous, that keep the person grounded in essential relationships and engaged with the world around him or her.

David Troxel joined the university in 1985. He and Virginia bonded almost immediately, realizing that the day center and their time spent with families could be a laboratory for learning, for themselves and others. Together, they could see the impact of the relationship-based approach and seek new ways to nurture connection and healing.

At the day center, staff and volunteers were called "Best Friends." Identifying the team in this way supported relationships and fought the isolation and fear that can come with dementia. It was also a catchy name that would appeal to their efforts to recruit more volunteers. They found that when a volunteer like Jane said, "Good morning, it's Jane, your Best Friend," the day center participant relaxed and smiled; the day was filled with activity and cooperation instead of struggle. Having a Best Friend proved comforting and helped to form connections.

The late Dr. William R. Markesbery, a neurologist whose research focused on the neuropathology of Alzheimer's, at the time was head of the University of Kentucky Alzheimer's Disease Research Center and had seen thousands of patients during his tenure. When he visited the Best Friends Day Center for the first time, he was stunned by the smiles, cooperation, and many ways in which his patients were participating. He was accustomed to hearing family tales of woe. Much to everyone's surprise, the serious-natured Dr. Markesbery danced with program participants, served ice cream cones, and participated in sing-alongs. He later said: "This center . . . it is the treatment for Alzheimer's."

To quote Oprah Winfrey, this was a "lightbulb" moment for us. Suddenly we understood that what a person with Alzheimer's disease or other dementias needs most is a *best friend*. We put this into practice in our day center program philosophy—engage the person as an individual, put the person before the task, know and use the person's Life Story, communicate effectively, and engage in fun and meaningful activity. What we learned formed the foundation for what is known as the Best Friends approach.

The Best Friends Day Center inspired our growing commitment to advocate for persons with dementia and for quality care. In 1988, the prestigious Robert Wood Johnson Foundation gave the program a major grant as part of its effort to encourage the development of adult day center care. We then began to write about our work. In a 1994 article, we first articulated and published our ideas in the form of an Alzheimer's Disease Bill of Rights, which in 2013 we updated and renamed the Best Friends™ Dementia Bill of Rights. In it, we took the then-uncommon stance that persons with dementia *do* have rights, and with the publication of the article, our approach began to gain widespread attention. In 1996, the first edition of *The Best Friends Approach to Alzheimer's Care* was published.

Initially, we worried that our book, with its optimistic and life-affirming view about the dementia journey, would be rejected by readers worn down by the losses and sadness that come with caring for loved ones with dementia. David wasn't sure whether the book would launch our careers or sink them. Virginia, more confident, thought we should say what we needed to say. Much to our relief and satisfaction, the book was an immediate success, and the Best Friends approach became a game-changer in the field of dementia care.

Readers told us how much the book meant to them. Ruth McReynolds, a woman with early-stage Alzheimer's, told us the book helped her become more accepting and optimistic about her future. Elayne Brill, a founder of the Alzheimer's Association in the greater San Francisco Bay Area and care partner for her husband, George, was initially reluctant to embrace the Best Friends philosophy. With time, however, "It all began to make sense. I never thought I'd say it, but you can come out on top," she said. Rita West Paustian thanked us for what became her father's bible as he cared for her mother: "I had often wondered how Dad seemed to know just how to engage my mother so that she continued to feel needed and loved. . . . He was putting Best Friends into practice. My mother's life, as well as ours, was enriched during that difficult time thanks to everything we learned about being a Best Friend."

Professionals in long-term care settings also took notice of our work. They saw that through the Best Friends approach, we were proposing a fundamental change in the culture of dementia care. "Best Friends started the shift in thinking away from the tasks of activities of daily living (ADLs) to the importance of the *way* we do them," says Linda Nickolisen, who worked for the state of Oregon in the 1990s as its Quality Resource Team Leader when it embraced Best Friends and created a statewide network of master trainers. "It was a rare thing to see state surveyors coming together with owners, administrators, and frontline staff, all embracing a new way of doing business. We loved the Best Friends philosophy because it drew attention to the fact that even our frailest and most needy elders deserved good care and valued relationships with staff and each other."

It was exciting to hear that a reader in South Africa, Michael Livni, had assigned each staff member in his nursing home to be a Best Friend to a resident and spend time each week one-on-one with the person. Michael wrote to us that this simple decision transformed care. We shared his idea in our book on staff training (*The Best Friends Staff*) and promoted it at conferences and workshops. Years later, Michael developed Alzheimer's disease himself and turned his experience into a well-regarded book, *The Japanese Therapists: Another Alzheimer's Autobiography*.

The successful statewide adoption of Best Friends in Oregon and the upsurge of interest in our book helped put the Best Friends approach on the map; however, not everyone was a convert. It was still common to encounter nurses in skilled settings who thought that their staff didn't have the time to be Best Friends and that the medical care of residents trumped everything else. Other professionals also thought that the Best Friends approach was too time consuming. Even in Oregon, where the Best Friends approach was supported at a very high level, it was a struggle to get everyone to embrace this new look at dementia care.

Changing the culture from a medical model (focusing on dementia as a set of symptoms needing medical and healthcare responses) to a social or relationship model (seeing how the environment and staff can enhance quality of life) was—and still is—a challenge. "It's a false construct to somehow talk about a social versus medical model—the Best Friends approach builds quality of life and meaning," says Wendy Schrag, Vice President of Clinical Services for Touchmark Retirement Communities and a nurse herself. "Shouldn't this be part of our best medical care?" Cynthia Lilly, who has worked in many residential dementia care settings and now serves as a Best Friends™ Expert Leader, agrees: "I argue that being kind, engaging, and knowing and using life stories in no way negates good medical care. In fact, when a nurse takes a few moments to make a friendship connection, the resident is more likely to take his or her medication."

Today, the Best Friends approach continues to change the culture of dementia care around the world.

We're very proud to be part of a movement that has helped launch incredible initiatives, such as The Eden Alternative® and The Green House® Project—innovative, life-affirming ideas that influence not only dementia care, but also elder care in general.

As of 2016, the Best Friends family of books have been published in various languages, including Spanish, Chinese (Mandarin), German,

Korean, Arabic, and Italian. The Dementia Bill of Rights (see Chapter 1) is also widely used internationally. Additional books in the Best Friends collection include *The Best Friends Staff: Building a Culture of Care in Alzheimer's Programs* and two volumes of *The Best Friends Book of Alzheimer's Activities,* written with Robin Hamon, Caregiver Support Coordinator at the Sanders Brown Center on Aging (University of Kentucky), and Tonya Cox, Administrator of The Homeplace at Midway for Christian Care Communities (Midway, Kentucky). As professional colleagues and continuing supporters and practitioners of the Best Friends approach, both Tonya (a Best Friends™ Expert Leader) and Robin have contributed their expertise to this new edition.

We are very gratified to see that many long-term care companies (small and large, for-profit and nonprofit) have been influenced by the Best Friends approach. Some have more formally adopted the principles by having staff attend the Best Friends™ Approach Institute for Master Trainer Certification, which equips them to train others within their care communities in Best Friends methods (for more information, visit http://bestfriends.healthpropress.com/).

Best Friends even made it to Hollywood! Actress Julianne Moore has a copy of *The Best Friends Approach to Alzheimer's Care* next to her laptop in the 2014 movie *Still Alice,* based on the book by Lisa Genova about a professor, wife, and mother with younger-onset dementia. When she won the Academy Award for her performance, she gracefully acknowledged the need for a greater focus on persons living with dementia and the importance of research to find a cure.

The first edition addressed both families and professional staff. This fully revised second edition continues to offer many ideas of value to family care partners. Its primary goal, however, is to focus more squarely on the concerns of professional care partners who work in-home or in a day center, residential, or other more formal care setting. It's designed to offer practical and easy-to-implement strategies for success as programs and communities adopt the Best Friends approach. Professional care partners, this book is for you!

At the time of this book's publication, it has been more than 10 years since the U.S. Food and Drug Administration has approved a new medication for Alzheimer's disease. The drug pipeline for the disease has seen disappointment after expensive disappointment. It turns out that the brain is quite a mystery, and solving the puzzle of Alzheimer's disease and other dementias isn't going to be easy. That's the bad news.

The good news is that there is a positive "treatment" available today in the form of the Best Friends approach. It will help you, your team, your in-home clients, day center participants, and residents create a caring community where music, arts, and exercise engage people with dementia and where morale is high, behaviors are managed with skill and confidence, and you can feel that you've made a difference every day you work as a Best Friend.

We want to express our gratitude to the many activity staff, program directors, CNAs, and other professional colleagues for consenting to be quoted in this edition. We're also grateful to everyone who gave us permission to share their stories, including persons with dementia and professionals working in the field of dementia care. One editorial choice we have consistently made since the first edition is to use full names, affiliations, and home towns, in order to add authenticity to our work and to fight the stigma that persons with dementia and their families can experience.

Finally, we'd like to get to know you. Please join our online community at www.facebook.com/bestfriendsapproach. We also invite you to visit our two websites, www.bestfriendsapproach.com and http://bestfriends.healthpropress.com.

Please join us in the journey.

Introduction

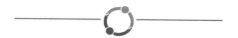

This second edition of *The Best Friends Approach to Dementia Care* is written for staff members who work in dementia care settings, including in-home, day centers, and residential care. It also addresses the concerns of readers who work in other types of service roles where they provide one-on-one therapy or work in other clinical and professional settings where people with dementia seek care, such as ambulance EMTs or the staff in an emergency room. Family care partners are encouraged to read the family edition of this book, *A Dignified Life: The Best Friends Approach to Dementia Care* (Bell & Troxel, 2012).

We have chosen not to include a chapter on Alzheimer's disease and other dementias because the Internet is a better source for learning about the rapidly changing information on diagnosis and treatment. Excellent websites, such as the U.S. Alzheimer's Association (www.alz.org), the National Institute on Aging Alzheimer's Disease Education and Referral Center (www.nia.nih.gov/alzheimers), and Alzheimer's Disease International (www.alz.co.uk), all offer accurate, reliable information on everything from the symptoms and stages of dementia to current research, clinical trials, and resources for care partners. See also the Appendix to this book, which includes recommended books, Web resources, and activity and programming resources.

Part 1 introduces you to the Best Friends philosophy—the concepts that are the foundation for becoming a Best Friends staff member. Part 2 shows how to apply the Best Friends™ approach to create a healing, therapeutic environment in your care setting, by learning and using the Life Story as you communicate and engage with your Best Friends. Part 3 presents tools you can use to begin adopting the Best Friends approach to transform your care setting's culture, including ways to overcome resistance to introducing the approach. You will also read accounts of how residential care communities have achieved great success by incorporating the Best Friends philosophy into their memory care programs.

Many of the core principles of the Best Friends approach have been summarized in display boxes appearing throughout this book. These can serve as useful reminders and training tools. They are therefore being made available to our readers as downloadable PDF files by visiting www.healthpropress.com/bell-downloads.

Notes on Terminology

The vocabulary of dementia care changes almost as quickly as research on the disease, so we want to define some key terms for you that you may be seeing used for the first time or in a new way.

We use the word *dementia* in the book's title and throughout the book as an umbrella term for any chronic disorder of the brain that causes forgetfulness, confusion, personality changes, language problems, and other challenges. Alzheimer's disease is the most common form of dementia, but there are many others. A good way of thinking about the differences is to think about automobiles. The word *automobile* or *car* describes a broad group (just like the word *dementia*). Under the heading of *cars* there are Toyotas, Volkswagens, Buicks, Hondas, and so forth (just as there are different types of dementia). Every Honda is a car, but not every car is a Honda. Similarly, every person with Alzheimer's disease has dementia, but not every person with dementia has Alzheimer's disease. The following "Dementia Umbrella" shows the various types of dementia (you can download a PDF of the figure from the Best Friends™ approach website www.healthpropress.com/bell-downloads).

The Best Friends approach will support you as you work with people living with any type of dementia. Even though the dementias are sometimes quite different—for example, people with Lewy body dementia often have profound hallucinations, and people with frontotemporal dementia have major personality changes—the key care techniques and strategies remain the same. (Specific strategies for engaging people with Lewy body dementia and frontotemporal dementia can be found in Chapters 5 and 7.)

In the first edition of this book, we italicized the phrase *person with dementia* or simply *person* to describe someone with Alzheimer's disease or other dementias. We wanted to remind readers that there is a person beneath the cloak of dementia, a person with a history, stories to tell,

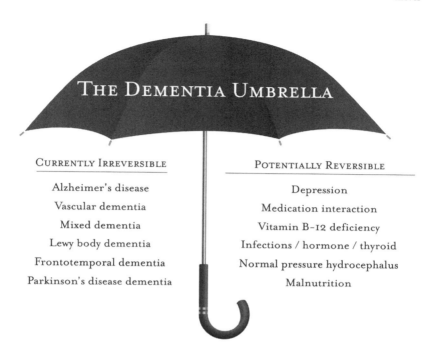

THE DEMENTIA UMBRELLA

CURRENTLY IRREVERSIBLE

Alzheimer's disease
Vascular dementia
Mixed dementia
Lewy body dementia
Frontotemporal dementia
Parkinson's disease dementia

POTENTIALLY REVERSIBLE

Depression
Medication interaction
Vitamin B-12 deficiency
Infections / hormone / thyroid
Normal pressure hydrocephalus
Malnutrition

feelings, and preferences who deserves dignified and loving care. We still believe that, and hope you do, too, but have dropped the practice in this edition.

Instead of *caregiver,* we use the term *care partner* to describe the family or staff member who is providing care and support. The traditional word *caregiver* has rich meaning to any of us who have provided support and care to a person with dementia, but it can imply a relationship where we do *for* the person instead of doing *with* the person.

We also believe *care partner* recognizes that the person with dementia still has much to offer, if given the opportunity. We understand that the partnership isn't always 50/50. For example, you may have to help the person quite a bit with personal care or medication management. The Best Friends approach will help you build cooperation so that care around activities of daily living (ADLs) is less of a struggle. ADLs such as bathing and other personal care tasks will be more successful, activities will see greater participation on the part of persons with dementia, and your day (and the person's day) will be more enjoyable and satisfying.

Another area where we have chosen to use more contemporary language is with respect to activities. As you will read in Chapter 6, the Best Friends approach asks you to reframe your traditional activity programming to be that of *engagement*, a concept that goes beyond the customary calendar of planned activities to also celebrate unplanned activities, some of which can be done in as little as 30 seconds.

Readers who appreciate correct grammar know that the pesky word *staff* can be singular or plural, which causes endless fits with our computer's grammar checker! Where we use the word *staff,* we treat it as plural rather than singular: "A Best Friends staff enjoys receiving praise for a job well done" instead of "A staff member enjoys receiving praise for a job well done."

The following are other key terms you will encounter as you read through the book:

Best Friends approach: A person-centered, compassionate approach grounded in the understanding that relationships are essential to dementia care. Incorporating into dementia care the elements of friendship—respect, empathy, support, trust, and humor—opens the doors to relationships that help persons living with dementia feel safe, secure, and valued and that also support family and professional care partners in navigating the dementia journey.

Dementia Bill of Rights: A summary of the rights of a person with dementia that can help shape improved plans of care as well as sensitivity to a person's needs (available as a downloadable PDF file at www.healthpropress.com/bell-downloads).

Best Friends Master Trainer: Someone who has received advanced instruction in the Best Friends approach and is certified to teach the approach to staff, colleagues, and volunteers in a care program. Master Trainer certification is conferred after a candidate demonstrates mastery of the principles and practices of the approach through the Best Friends Approach Institute for Master Trainer Certification. For more information, contact bestfriends@healthpropress.com.

Knack: The art of doing difficult things with ease by using clever tricks and strategies that help care partners become less task oriented and more relationship centered. (A downloadable PDF file featuring the Elements of Knack is available at www.healthpropress.com/bell-downloads.)

Life Story: A summary of the key elements of a person's life that is gathered from family, friends, and the person and that can be used to personalize care in daily situations. By learning details of the person's past, you can improve communication, shape successful activities, and provide important cues that help make life smoother.

Recasting relationships from staff to Best Friend: In a care community, the process of replacing clinical, task-focused language in day-to-day responsibilities and job descriptions with the language of friendship helps to foster authentic relationships that effectively help people with dementia feel safe, secure, and valued.

Therapeutic environment: We often think of an environment as sofas and chairs, lighting, and art. Although there is rich literature about good design for dementia care, the environment also includes people and programs. A therapeutic or healing environment is based on real knowledge of the history, preferences, and pastimes of the person with dementia; involves communicating with the person in ways that affirm and respect; and offers activities, planned and spontaneous, that keep the person grounded in essential relationships and engaged with the world around him or her.

To the many professional care partners around the world who
support persons with Alzheimer's disease and other dementias
and who have inspired us with their hard work and loving spirit.

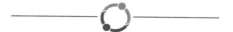

*"I dislike social workers, nurses, and friends
who do not treat me as a real person."*

—Rebecca Riley

PART 1

The Best Friends™ Approach

For those of you who are familiar with the books and have attended workshops and conferences on the Best Friends™ approach, this section's many new ideas, language, and stories will inspire you to keep up your important work to change the culture of care in your care setting. Even great friendships need nurturing, and the opening chapters offer you a thorough Best Friends "tune-up."

For readers who are new to Best Friends, this section will inspire you to learn and use the approach. You are probably already doing some of the things we suggest, since so many staff working in dementia care are motivated by the heart. If reading this section leaves you concerned about mistakes in the past, please don't dwell on them or beat yourself up. As you move through these opening chapters, you'll find that our intuitive, easy-to-learn approach will profoundly shape your work style going forward.

This section begins with the Life Story of Rebecca Riley, who was one of Virginia Bell's oldest friends and a person with younger-onset Alzheimer's disease who influenced our early work at the Best Friends™ Day Center.

Let's meet Rebecca Riley.

CHAPTER 1

Starting with the Person

The Life Story and Human Rights

The Best Friends™ approach has been shaped by real people—people with dementia we have been privileged to meet and work with over the years. One of our earliest and most important "teachers" was a college friend of Virginia Bell. Rebecca Riley was a nurse educator who was diagnosed with Alzheimer's disease in her 50s. As she traveled what we now call the continuum of care—from home care, to day center care, to residential care—we were happy to share almost all of the dementia journey with her, including hundreds of hours spent together at the Best Friends™ Day Center.

Being a Best Friends care partner to Rebecca came very naturally to Virginia because the two women already were friends. The strong relationship between them was a starting point for a long journey. Even during rough moments, Virginia and Rebecca were able to draw on their long-term friendship.

You can't be a friend without knowing details of someone's life. Other members of the Best Friends™ Day Center staff were able to draw on a very useful document: Rebecca's Life Story. Knowing a person's Life Story is a key concept of the Best Friends approach, as you will see, and we will allude to Rebecca's Life Story many times throughout this book. (See Chapter 3 for a detailed discussion of how to prepare and use the Life Story.)

Although Rebecca died many years ago, she lives on as a symbol of strength and courage throughout this book. We want to introduce you to Rebecca because we learned much from her that has helped us shape the life-affirming and successful philosophy you will learn about from this book. Let's meet one of our first Best Friends through her Life Story, as told to us by Rebecca and her husband, Jo.

Life Story of Rebecca Matheny Riley

Rebecca was born January 8, 1925, to Elsie Arnold and S. F. Matheny. She was the first granddaughter on both sides of her family. Rebecca and her only sister, Mary Frances, 18 months younger, were very close as children. Her grandmother came to this country in 1892 from Austria, where some of her family still resides. When Rebecca was only 3 years old, her mother died, and her grandparents became parents to Rebecca and her little sister.

Rebecca adored her grandparents. She and her sister were happy-go-lucky as they played in the creek that ran through their grandparents' farm. Catching frogs and tadpoles that lived in the creek was a favorite pastime on a hot summer day. On autumn days, they enjoyed gathering hickory nuts and walnuts that had fallen from the many trees on the farm.

Grandpa had lots of animals, including one horse that he allowed the little girls to ride alone. This horse was very slow and deliberate and always dependable as he carried the girls safely on his back. One day, this trusty horse became frightened. As he galloped faster and faster, the girls held on for dear life. Rebecca remembered the scary ride and how happy she and her sister were when a neighbor rescued them.

Rebecca had many friends at school. A favorite game to play with her classmates was hide-and-seek. When Rebecca was in the first grade, she invited her entire class to come home with her after school. This was a big surprise to Grandpa and Grandma. Although they all had a great time playing at the farm, she remembers a serious discussion about asking permission before inviting so many friends to visit.

Rebecca and Mary Frances were often responsible for doing the dishes after supper to help their grandmother. They argued about whose turn it was to clean up the kitchen.

Rebecca's father remarried, and she soon had two brothers, Sam and Earl. As Rebecca grew older, she wondered about her mother: "What was she really like?" "Why did she have to leave me when I was such a little girl?" Although Grandma and Grandpa were wonderful "parents," Rebecca often had sad thoughts about not knowing her mother.

Even as a young girl, Rebecca was goal oriented. She had a determined spirit and a mind of her own and refused to take "no" for an answer. That spirit remained very much a part of her. She always wanted to be helpful, especially to others in great need. She was motivated to learn, making her an excellent student.

During her youth, Rebecca was a member of the Methodist church and active in the Epworth League sponsored by the church. Her religious faith fed her spirit and desire to be helpful. She often made known her life goals: to be a nurse, serve as a missionary, and marry a minister.

During her years at Stanford High School, Rebecca played in the band. She was also a member of the Girl's Reserve Club and graduated with honors. After graduation, she enrolled in nurse training at Good Samaritan Hospital in Lexington, Kentucky. As a nursing student she met her husband while he was a patient in the hospital. Although nursing students at that time were not allowed to remain in school after marriage, Rebecca relied on her determined spirit and became the first married nursing student at the hospital.

On April 20, 1945, she married Jo M. Riley, an ordained minister in the Christian Church (Disciples of Christ). His pastorates took them to Kokomo, Indiana; Wilson, North Carolina; Decatur, Illinois; Louisville, Kentucky; and Centralia, Illinois. She taught church classes for children and young adults and was very supportive of all church activities. She served on a national Week of Compassion committee for her church. This was a special honor for Rebecca, giving her the opportunity to use her expertise on a national level.

Rebecca was nominated Mother of the Year while living in Kokomo, Indiana, and was the president of the Minister's Wives Organization of Illinois. These honors were very special to her. The community also benefited from Rebecca's helping hands. She was a Girl Scout leader for several years.

Rebecca and Jo were parents to three children, Lucinda, Joetta, and Louis, and grandparents to Josh, Ian, Tristan, and Grant. Rebecca had always been family oriented; her family came first.

Rebecca and Jo owned a cottage on Crystal Lake in Michigan. Each summer the family vacationed there. Given an hour's notice, Rebecca said they could be packed up and ready to go. This was a wonderful place for the children to play. The cottage was located just a stone's throw from

The life story can be supplemented with photographs of the person. At right, Rebecca is pictured from her childhood (seen here with her younger sister, Mary Frances), through her early nursing career, her marriage to Jo, and her young adulthood, raising a family.

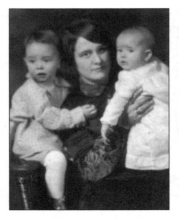

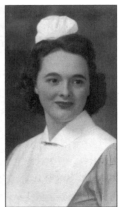

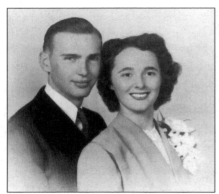

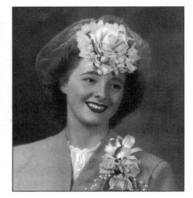

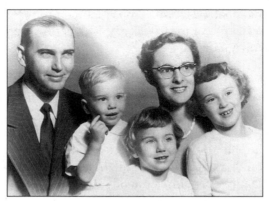

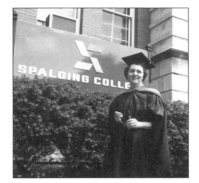

Rebecca graduated with a master's in nursing education. As her dementia progressed, she found comfort in playing with her dogs and traveling with Jo. Even when she required continuous care at a facility, she still had her soft eyes and warm smile.

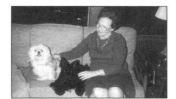

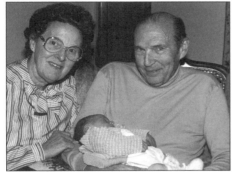

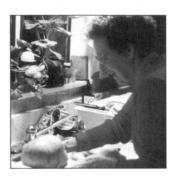

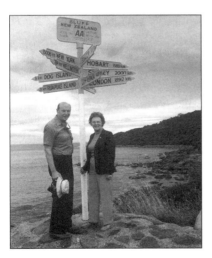

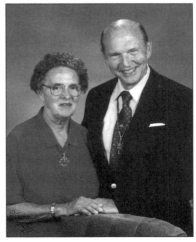

the water. Swimming and enjoying their rowboat were great ways for the family to spend time together. Also, family and friends returned each year to nearby cottages. Often, these friends gathered with the Riley family for picnics at special locations along the lake. One of Rebecca's favorite activities was a breakfast picnic on a hot summer day. The sand dunes nearby were very tall and inviting to climb after a picnic.

Cooking was an art for Rebecca. Wherever she lived, she learned how to prepare local dishes and delighted in serving them to visitors to the community. Two of Rebecca's specialties were "popcorn" cake and persimmon pudding. Rebecca remembers preparing a reception for 500 people—what a big task!

In 1972, Rebecca returned to school to earn a bachelor of science in nursing, and in 1974 she received a master's in education from Spaulding College. She taught nursing students until she was diagnosed with Alzheimer's in July 1984. Spaulding College, Jefferson Community College, and Centralia College all benefited from her gift of teaching.

After their children were grown, Jo and Rebecca traveled to England, Scotland, Australia, New Zealand, Israel, Jordan, China, Russia, Austria, and other European countries. While in Austria, they visited Rebecca's grandmother's home, the fulfillment of a dream for Rebecca.

Rebecca enjoyed classical music, knitting, sewing, reading, and homemaking. Her favorite hymn was *Amazing Grace*. Her dog, Corky, was a constant companion, especially after her diagnosis of Alzheimer's disease. Corky reminded her of her childhood pet dog, Briar.

When Rebecca was diagnosed with Alzheimer's, she openly and honestly shared her feelings about the disease for as long as she was able to do so. Rebecca wanted to do everything she could to be of help to others.

Woven through all of her roles in life is a common thread: Rebecca was always a teacher. She probably did her best teaching after she was diagnosed with Alzheimer's. Rebecca was determined to make a difference. She enrolled in research studies to help find a cause for the disease, and she taught everyone who would listen what it's like to live with Alzheimer's.

What Rebecca Taught Us

Rebecca was an important early participant in the Best Friends™ Day Center, because she could express her needs and concerns—early on through her words and writing, later with her actions and feelings. As we spent time with her and listened and responded, she helped us develop our working ideas, particularly when we were able to turn her anxiety into feelings of calm or her tears into laughter.

What we learned from her early years with us was integral to the development of the Best Friends approach, including that:

- *We are more than just our memory and cognition.* Despite profound losses, there was still a person there with likes and dislikes, opinions and feelings.

- *Each person with Alzheimer's is a unique individual.* As Virginia likes to say, "When you've met one person with Alzheimer's, you've met one person with Alzheimer's." In a moment you'll learn how the desire to honor individuals and their rights became the starting point of our Best Friends™ Dementia Bill of Rights.

- *Life Story matters.* From her family's diligent efforts to provide Life Story information and from her long history with Virginia, we know so much about Rebecca. When she was having a bad day, we would "dip into the reservoir" and come up with just the right story, topic, question, or activity that pleased her.

- *Empathy is important.* Even when Rebecca had angry moments, we recognized that it was the disease talking, not something we should take personally. The behavior was caused by the symptoms of dementia, not because Rebecca was being deliberately mean.

- *Productive and interesting activities keep people connected and engaged in life.* At the day center, Rebecca gravitated toward more adult and purposeful activities, particularly ones that involved helping others. She also valued the unstructured times when she could share smiles, hugs, and short conversations and even just sit out in the garden watching the world go by.

- *Communicate, communicate, communicate.* Even when her language skills began to falter, Rebecca loved when our day center staff and volunteers would ask for her opinion, talk to her about the day, and communicate with her nonverbally through lots of hugs and smiles.

- *Stages of dementia can be arbitrary and limiting.* Families and persons with dementia want a general understanding of the overall spectrum of dementia and their place in it. Although staging can be a valuable tool for clinicians or research trials, we realized that Rebecca and other Day Center participants supposedly in the same stage of the disease process had different personalities, strengths, and abilities. Rather than focusing on stages, we focused on each individual and his or her own unique journey.

- *In many ways, socialization is the treatment for dementia.* Dementia is a disease of isolation. Little by little, persons with dementia step away from—or are excluded from—the world around them. Rebecca felt less alone at the fun-filled, relationship-centered day program where volunteers and staff provided her with love and friendship.

Rebecca Riley was a successful, motivated woman full of life and concern for others. One can imagine that her diagnosis of Alzheimer's disease must have been shocking. For someone who was always purposeful and organized, the confusion and forgetfulness that come with dementia must have been highly frustrating. There were days when she must have been angry at the world and fearful about her future.

As a staff member working with older adults, you have probably met people like Rebecca—the person who has long been considered a brilliant lawyer, dedicated mom, or caring grandmother but who now struggles to put on a sweater or participate in a simple word game. How can you address her frustration and anger when confusion and forgetfulness happen? How can you encourage her to take part in activities and be a part of life? How can you help her feel safe, secure, and valued? How can you support her basic rights?

The answer is to focus on the person, not the task. The core of the Best Friends approach is simple: *Treat the person with dementia as if he or she is a Best Friend.* Like a friend, bring your knowledge of his or her Life Story and personal quirks and preferences to every interaction. Communicate sensitively, engage in fun and meaningful activities together, and try to bring out the best in the person instead of merely "managing" his or her disease. Use the idea of friendship to build a relationship and connection and to help the person overcome the isolation and fear that can accompany dementia.

In Rebecca's case, being her Best Friend meant treating her with respect, communicating with her, encouraging her, giving her simple chores and jobs, and reminding her about her many accomplishments. In short, we recognized that she was much, much more than her diagnosis—a core concept of the Best Friends approach!

The Best Friends Dementia Bill of Rights

The early 1990s, when Rebecca and her family were on the dementia journey, were challenging times for family and professional care

In Their Shoes

Imagine that you have just been asked to be Rebecca's care partner. What do you think would be important to her each day? Here are some possibilities:

- Recognize her as a nurse.
- Ask her for her opinion.
- Encourage her to teach a simple class on knitting.
- Ask about her husband, Jo, and their children.
- Reminisce about her time at Crystal Lake.
- Celebrate a tradition of her faith.
- Cook one of her favorite dishes together.

What former nurses have you been a care partner to in your dementia program? It's likely that they have been organized, committed to helping others, used to having some authority, knowledgeable about healthcare and medicine, and generally productive people. What are some ways you can engage with them or honor their past profession?

partners. Yes, public awareness of dementia was growing, and new programs and services were springing up. Yet few understood and embraced the idea that a therapeutic environment could lead to a better life for persons with dementia. Even more discouraging, few recognized that underneath the cloak of dementia there was still a person, someone who deserves our best care and support and who has the right to live with choice and dignity. Too often, the disease got more attention and respect than the person.

Because of our friendships with people like Rebecca, we knew that regardless of the diagnosis, a person with dementia was a full-fledged human being. Because we knew their histories and what sparked laughter and what triggered tears, we knew they were people who deserved to be treated well. We weren't just being nice! We firmly believed that they had the *right* to be treated well.

In an effort to raise the bar for dementia care, we published in 1994 "An Alzheimer's Disease Bill of Rights" in the *American Journal of Alzheimer's Care and Related Disorders and Research*. It featured a 12-point list that was quickly adopted by forward-looking organizations and care partners, not just in the United States but around the world.

Lilia Mendoza, Ph.D., one of Mexico's leaders in the field of Alzheimer's, noted that this was the first time anyone had viewed dementia care from a human rights perspective. Although the Alzheimer's Disease Bill of Rights had no force of law, the concept gained traction, and it was reprinted by groups such as Alzheimer's Disease International (in the journal *Global Perspective* [(1995, February/March), 6(1), 11]), and by local and international Alzheimer's associations and societies. The Bill of Rights also caught the attention of long-term care program staff, who viewed it as a foundational document for assessing and improving their own dementia programs. Copies of the Bill of Rights, translated into many different languages, appeared as posters and handouts in long-term care programs and offices around the world.

Over time, many of the once-controversial planks of the Bill of Rights—such as the idea that people have a right to be informed of their diagnosis—had become accepted practices. Others, such as the right to be free, whenever possible, of psychotropic medications, had launched discussions and searches for alternatives that continue to grow.

For this edition, this influential document was updated to reflect the progress in the care and understanding of those living with dementia. We changed its name to the Dementia Bill of Rights to reflect the growing awareness that Alzheimer's disease, although the most common, is not the only type of dementia. A high-quality dementia care program must provide training for its team on each type of dementia so that staff can, for example, understand the experience of a person with Lewy body dementia or frontotemporal dementia as well as that of a person with a classic presentation of Alzheimer's disease.

Dementia Bill of Rights

The rights of persons with dementia are at the very core of the Best Friends approach. As a Best Friends care partner, please commit yourself to understanding and respecting these rights so that you, too, will make them the centerpiece of your approach to care. We encourage you to download and print copies of the Dementia Bill of Rights to share with your team. They can be a source for staff and family education, a checklist to gauge your program's success, and a foundational document for delivering high-quality dementia care.

Let's look at each principle of the Dementia Bill of Rights (Figure 1.1).

DEMENTIA BILL of RIGHTS

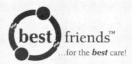

*...for the **best** care!*

Every person diagnosed with Alzheimer's disease or other dementia deserves:

- To be informed of one's diagnosis
- To have appropriate, ongoing medical care
- To be treated as an adult, listened to, and afforded respect for one's feelings and point of view
- To be with individuals who know one's life story, including cultural and spiritual traditions
- To experience meaningful engagement throughout the day
- To live in a safe and stimulating environment
- To be outdoors on a regular basis
- To be free from psychotropic medications whenever possible
- To have welcomed physical contact, including hugging, caressing, and handholding
- To be an advocate for oneself and for others
- To be part of a local, global, or online community
- To have care partners well trained in dementia care

Figure 1.1. The Best Friends™ Dementia Bill of Rights, by Virginia Bell and David Troxel. Copyright © 2013 by Health Professions Press, Inc. All rights reserved. www.healthpropress/alzbill

The Right to Be Informed of One's Diagnosis

Almost all physicians believe that ethical practice demands that they inform patients of a serious medical diagnosis, even against family wishes. Understanding one's diagnosis allows the person to have a voice in his or her treatment and to make important decisions about the use of services, finances, estate planning, and end-of-life care.

As people concerned about their memory consult their physicians and receive diagnoses much earlier, doctors are putting the diagnosis into the broader context of the patient's life. Encouraging the person to exercise, listen to music, volunteer, and socialize—to stay active in the flow of life—reinforces the idea that persons with dementia are more than their diagnosis. And that is a concept that Best Friends care partners live and care by.

The Right to Have Appropriate, Ongoing Medical Care

Persons with dementia and their families often struggle to find appropriate, ongoing care from physicians who are knowledgeable about the disease. Families tell us that even today, it's hard to find a good, caring physician or medical team.

Hopefully your program has good nursing support and relationships with medical advisors who are knowledgeable about medications, because some medications and combinations of medications can impair cognition or have other negative side effects. Good medical care and oversight also help control "excess disabilities," such as urinary tract infections, pain, and depression. A capable and caring neurologist or other physician who is willing to discuss concerns and needs can also help your team and your families navigate the journey, including with respect to end-of-life advice and care.

The Right to Be Treated as an Adult, Listened to, and Afforded Respect for One's Feelings and Point of View

The person has led a full life, rich in experiences. Even late into the illness, the person will retain a sense of her personal history, achievements, and values. Activities and language should be age appropriate and meaningful. Be sure that you aren't asking a former federal judge to cut out paper dolls. People in their 70s should not be spoken to as if they were 7 years old.

Respecting adulthood also means being present for the person, actively listening and working to make the communication connection. When words fail, we can respond to the person's feelings and emotions.

Responding with just the right words of friendship, a smile, or a hug can make the difference between a day of strife and a day of success.

Persons with dementia still have a point of view, and offering simple choices, respecting past traditions, and honoring present preferences can all help the person feel more in control of his or her life as well as build self-esteem.

The Right to Be with Individuals Who Know One's Life Story, Including Cultural and Spiritual Traditions

Knowing a person's Life Story and traditions is an essential part of excellent dementia care. The person feels secure and affirmed when his or her identity is acknowledged and preferences are honored. When staff members know that a resident loves coffee with cream and sugar, once served as the local mayor, or is a retired firefighter, they can use this information to offer compliments, reminisce, break the ice before personal care, or redirect the person with skill and confidence.

Cultural traditions have deep roots that often survive well into a person's journey with dementia. Does the person come from an African American community where elders are treated with great respect (is it important to call the person Mr. or Mrs. Thompson instead of addressing the person in a more familiar way by using his or her first name)? Does the person come from a family tradition of loud, boisterous, food-filled dinners or from a tradition that is more reserved? Knowing these family and cultural traditions helps avoid mistakes and ensures more sensitive and supportive care.

It's also a good idea to be aware of spiritual traditions. Has the person belonged to a specific faith community, enjoyed religious music, used rosary beads, or enjoyed daily prayers? Does he or she find a spiritual connection through nature or the arts? When we know these traditions, we can help the person remain connected to faith and spiritual practices.

The Right to Experience Meaningful Engagement Throughout the Day

A day that involves conversation, stimulates the senses, promotes new information and learning, celebrates music, encourages outdoor time, and includes group and individualized activities helps the person feel safe, secure, and valued. Exercise is particularly important, and evidence continues to grow that it's good not only for the body but also for the brain.

A fundamental principle of human rights is involvement in the community. The best memory care programs keep the person engaged by visiting the local museum or attending sports and recreational events, concerts, and school programs.

The Right to Live in a Safe and Stimulating Environment

Whether it's a home setting or a long-term care community, the living environment should be designed around the needs of the person. It should be safe, well lit, uncluttered, and pleasant and offer areas for walking. The environment should also be stimulating and include music, the smell of freshly baked bread or good food, and furniture that encourages socialization.

Twenty years ago, we believed that structure and routine were essential. Today we know that just as consistency is valuable, so is mixing it up and trying new things. We've learned that persons with dementia are more resilient than we thought and enjoy a sense of novelty.

The Right to Be Outdoors on a Regular Basis

Fresh air and sunshine are important! Just feeling warm sunshine can boost morale, stimulate the senses, provide natural vitamin D, and promote a good night's sleep. Being outdoors can also lead to pleasant activities, such as enjoying flowers and bird or people watching.

Outdoor activity is particularly important for people in residential programs where most activities occur indoors. Consider encouraging outdoor chores, such as sweeping, raking, filling bird feeders, or tending to a raised flowerbed or vegetable garden. Get residents outside whenever possible to connect them with nature and fight depression. It's never too late to enjoy a hummingbird or rainbow.

The Right to Be Free from Psychotropic Medications Whenever Possible

Psychotropic drugs can improve behavior, but they come with potentially dangerous side effects, such as an increased risk of falls, urinary tract infections, skin problems, and (in the case of atypical antipsychotics) a higher risk of death.

It's also hard to make the choice of medication and dosage correctly, particularly for fragile people in their 80s and older. In his book *Dementia Beyond Drugs: Changing the Culture of Care* (2010), Geriatrician

Dr. G. Allen Power suggests that even at their best, psychotropic medications generally work only 20% of the time.

Instead of immediately opting for medication, look first at the environment, activity and engagement program, staff training, and individual situation. As Chapter 7 will show, behavior that is challenging for staff can be addressed with techniques from the Best Friends philosophy. For example, distrust and suspicion, which care partners often label as paranoia, might be reduced by enhanced lighting, more exercise, and skillful redirection. A person may be less combative in the shower when you take your time, smile, and use his or her Life Story.

A sedated life is not a good life, and when a person experiences added confusion caused by medication, you may be exchanging one set of problems for another. Avoid psychotropic drugs when possible and remember that hugs are generally better than drugs!

The Right to Have Welcomed Physical Contact, Including Hugging, Caressing, and Hand-Holding

Persons with dementia benefit from touch and intimacy, and we should, with permission, offer a friendly handshake, pat on the back, hand massage, or hug. Offering this physical contact helps a person feel connected to others, can be reassuring to someone who is anxious, and can bring particular comfort to a person in late dementia.

Thoughtful professionals who write and speak about sexuality and dementia think that although it's important to protect the person's right to intimacy, persons with dementia may not be able to give informed consent. Inclusive and thoughtful care planning involving the person, staff, and family supports a wise and successful outcome. You'll find much more on this controversial topic in Chapter 7.

The Right to Be an Advocate for Oneself and for Others

When the original Alzheimer's Disease Bill of Rights was published, it was rare to see persons with dementia writing and speaking out about their situation. Today, they serve on boards, connect with others on the Internet, write, and share their stories and points of view at Alzheimer's conferences.

Advocating for themselves and others, they are adding meaning to their lives while helping others who do not have a voice. They are raising money for research, advocating for better medical care and new medications, creating local early-stage support groups, and supporting services for their care partners and themselves. They are making a difference and feeling *empowered*—not a word one usually associates with dementia!

Honoring and facilitating a person's advocacy is another manifestation of the core Best Friends value: that persons with dementia at home, in day centers, and in residential care should have as much say about their life as possible. As a Best Friends care partner, you support this right every time you slow down, listen carefully, and respect a person's wishes. All of us want to have a voice.

The Right to Be Part of a Local, Global, or Online Community

Most persons with dementia want to help others and feel connected to their communities. Attending a church social, going to the local farmer's market, enjoying a concert, phoning the grandchildren on Skype, reading a hometown paper online, or enjoying a local sporting event help the person to feel and be a part of life both locally and in the world at large.

Wi-Fi, computers, and smartphones make it easy to stay connected. Many people enjoy surfing the Internet to see pictures of their family members, friends, and hometowns; read up on a favorite subject; watch a YouTube video, T.V. show, or movie; or even be a part of an online support group.

As part of a very positive trend, many long-term care programs are developing civic engagement programs, such as making dog biscuits for the local animal shelter, writing letters to troops, or crafting a gift for children, all of which creates a sense of purpose for people with dementia (and for all of us, too).

The Right to Have Care Partners Well Trained in Dementia Care

With Alzheimer's disease and other dementias in the news every day and with so much information available through the media, websites, blogs, workshops, and conferences, there is no excuse for professional programs to provide poor care to persons with dementia.

The consumer is also getting smarter and knows a good dementia care program from a not-so-good program. The market will reward companies and organizations that do a good job of training and supporting staff, creating dementia-friendly environments, and offering robust engagement programs.

When family and professional care partners are well informed, they not only provide better care, but also feel more fulfilled by a job well done.

The Dementia Bill of Rights Working for You

How can you apply the Dementia Bill of Rights to your work? Think about one person you have built a relationship with as a care partner. Now read through the Dementia Bill of Rights item by item with this person in mind. How are you doing?

We used Rebecca Riley as our person, and here's what we found:

- To be informed of one's diagnosis
  - *Rebecca wanted to know her situation and was happy to be asked to keep a diary of her experiences and participate in education and training programs.*
- To have appropriate, ongoing medical care
  - *Rebecca's family was assured that she had good medical care, including support from a university memory disorder clinic.*
- To be treated as an adult, listened to, and afforded respect for one's feelings and point of view
  - *We were careful to engage with Rebecca as an adult, giving her simple but meaningful choices and taking time to listen to her, even after her words began to fail her.*
- To be with individuals who know one's Life Story, including cultural and spiritual traditions
  - *We strived to know and use Rebecca's Life Story throughout the day.*
- To experience meaningful engagement throughout the day
  - *No crayons for Rebecca! She enjoyed discussions about the arts, family, and religion.*
- To live in a safe and stimulating environment
  - *Rebecca thrived at the Best Friends™ Day Center, and her family was also very engaged.*
- To be outdoors on a regular basis
  - *Daily walks lifted Rebecca's spirits.*
- To be free from psychotropic medications whenever possible
  - *Rebecca was able to enjoy life without psychotropic medications.*
- To have welcomed physical contact, including hugging, caressing, and hand-holding
  - *She loved the simple act of holding hands.*

Continued

- To be an advocate for oneself and for others
  - *Rebecca participated in dementia conferences.*
- To be part of a local, global, or online community
  - *Rebecca kept up with many friends and regularly participated in her faith community.*
- To have care partners well trained in dementia care
  - *Rebecca benefited from being in a model day program. Later, her residential care program embraced the Best Friends philosophy with good staff training.*

Conclusion

It's striking how well Rebecca Riley and many other early participants did in the Best Friends™ Day Center program. Several families had reported that "mother was impossible" or "she won't do anything," or, worse, that the person with dementia was hostile and combative. Yet as we developed our day program and the Best Friends approach, we were able to turn failures into successes, all because we were willing to develop authentic relationships, treat them with respect, and recognize that they were much, much more than their diagnosis. What we learned from participants like Rebecca became the building blocks for the Best Friends approach, which Chapter 2 will outline.

The Dementia Bill of Rights captures the essence of the Best Friends approach by focusing on the needs of the individual. Individuals, families, and professionals who adopt best practices that respect these rights will find that the result is an improved plan of care and increased sensitivity to the needs of a person with dementia, wherever that person is in the progression of the disease.

CHAPTER 2

Introducing the
Best Friends Approach

We'd like for you to consider the following two scenarios. As you read them, we think you'll begin to see how persons with dementia have many of the same needs that we do and how being a Best Friend can be a powerful tool for supporting quality of life.

Scenario 1

Imagine meeting an old friend for lunch and finding your normally upbeat, positive friend in tears. As a friend, how would you respond? You would probably:

- *Ask her what is wrong.* (Try to get more information. She tells you that she has been laid off from a job that she loved and is worried about her financial future.)
- *Show you understand and have empathy.* (Let her know that this has happened to you and that her feelings of worry and disappointment are okay.)
- *Affirm her feelings.* ("It's really terrible that they treated you that way. No wonder you are upset.")
- *Listen.* (Focus, nod your head, take time to hear her.)
- *Give a compliment.* ("You are so talented and the best salesperson.")
- *Be encouraging.* ("The job market is strong right now. I'm sure you'll get some offers and maybe even make more money!")

- *Offer a hug.* (Do so only if you know she likes to be touched.)
- *Use your sense of humor.* ("You always told me you were tired of the travel. Now you can stay home and watch *Dancing with the Stars* with us while we try out the newest cocktails!")
- *And, finally, change the mood, in this case with a favorite dessert.* ("Let me treat you to that brownie sundae you love, with some extra whipped cream. Now is the time for chocolate!")

Your friend thanks you for your support, stops sobbing, laughs, and asks if you know any sales executives. By the last bite, you have truly been there for your friend. You've shown your support and cheered her up.

Scenario 2

Imagine a similar scenario in your memory care program. A resident who is normally calm and cheerful is sitting in her chair sobbing. As a Best Friends care partner, what should you do? You might:

- *Ask her what is wrong.* (Try to get more information. Even though you know that her son visited this morning, she says she has not seen him in a long time, and she is worried about him.)
- *Show you understand and have empathy.* (Think about how you would feel if a child of yours didn't visit you for a long time.)
- *Affirm her feelings.* ("No wonder you are feeling so sad!")
- *Listen.* (Slow down, make eye contact, nod your head.)
- *Give a compliment.* ("You are the best mom.")
- *Be encouraging.* ("I'm sure he will be visiting soon. Let's try his cell phone.")
- *Offer a hug.* (Do so only if you know the person likes to be touched.)
- *Use your sense of humor.* ("That son of yours is such a funny character. You are going to have to set him straight the next time he comes!")
- *And, finally, change the mood or redirect, in this case with a favorite dessert.* ("Let me treat you to your favorite chocolate ice cream with lots of whipped cream. Now is the time for chocolate!")

The resident relaxes, smiles, and begins talking about how proud she is of her son's accomplishments.

It's remarkable that in these two scenarios your approach with your friend over lunch is the same approach you can take with the resident. Both the old friend and resident need a Best Friend to show understanding and empathy, to listen, and to cheer them up. Persons with dementia have all of the same needs that we all have. By engaging with them as friends, we can actually redirect and change sadness to happiness, fear to contentment. Friendship and empathy can transform the way persons with dementia feel and behave.

Just like our friend who lost her job, all of us have moments such as those listed in the left column of Figure 2.1. Using Best Friends strategies to show you understand and care, you may be able to move a person from the feelings in the left column to the more positive states of mind in the right column, even if just for a few moments. Those moments add up. Like pearls on a string, these moments begin to create, piece by piece, pearl by pearl, something beautiful. And that's the goal of the Best Friends™ approach!

You can see the approach in action in the following cartoon strip (see Figure 2.2). The first page shows a residential care community where staff members are good people and well intentioned, but focus on tasks more than the residents, who aren't particularly engaged in

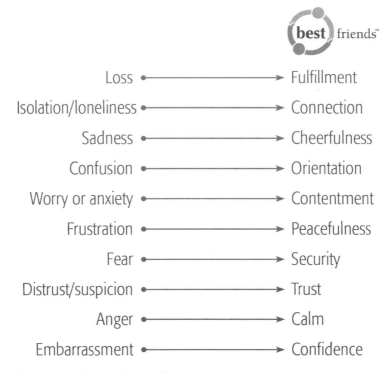

Figure 2.1. Moving the needle.

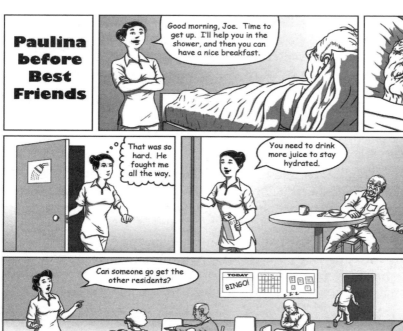

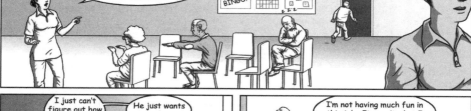

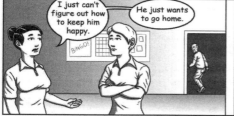

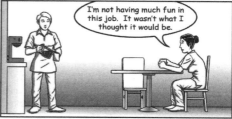

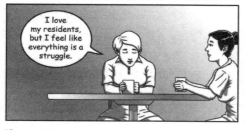

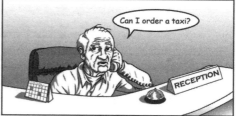

Figure 2.2.

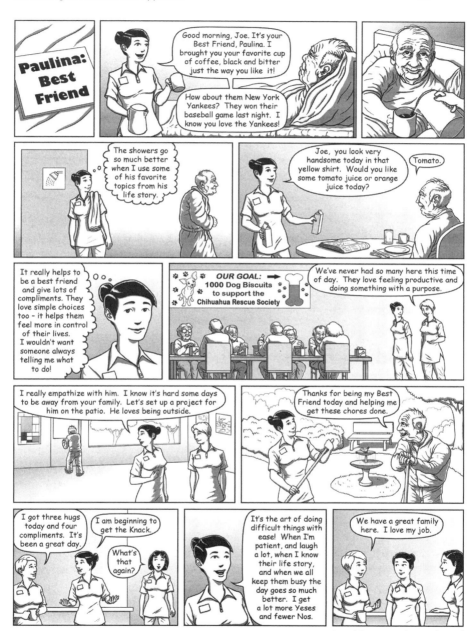

Figure 2.2. *(continued)*

activities. Staff members struggle to find success (and meaning) in their work. Unfortunately, this is still very common.

Now look at the second page of the cartoon. The community and its staff embrace the Best Friends approach, know and use the Life Story, create an interesting day, and foster relationships. Residents are engaged and happy, and staff members experience more success.

Consider our friend Rebecca Riley. If an aide who didn't know much about Rebecca entered her room to help her get dressed, even the gentle-spirited Rebecca might have told the aide to go away. That same care partner, now trained in the Best Friends approach, enters with a friendly smile and some simple questions about Rebecca's life as a nurse. Feeling a sense of connection and trust to the staff member, Rebecca now cooperates with personal care. What might have taken 45 minutes of struggle now takes 20 minutes or less. The Best Friends approach actually saves time.

Putting the person before the task, knowing and using the Life Story, communicating effectively, and engaging in fun and meaningful activity form the foundation of the Best Friends approach. Let's take a look at the specific building blocks that are a part of that foundation.

Building Blocks of the Best Friends Approach

Seven basic building blocks form the Best Friends approach, beginning with the affirmation that even people who are cognitively compromised have inherent rights. Good care and quality of life are human rights issues. By valuing and honoring the rights of persons with dementia, the Best Friends approach seeks to move the culture of dementia care *away* from stigma and failure and *toward* acceptance and success.

Throughout this book, we explore the many nuances of creating and nurturing relationships that bring out the best in a person with dementia, reduce behavior that is challenging, foster cooperation, and evoke embedded social graces and manners. Understanding each building block can help you learn to see persons with dementia differently as you begin to implement a Best Friends approach in your work:

- Recognize the basic rights of a person with dementia.
- Understand what it's like to have dementia.
- Know and use the person's Life Story.
- Know just what to say when communication is breaking down.

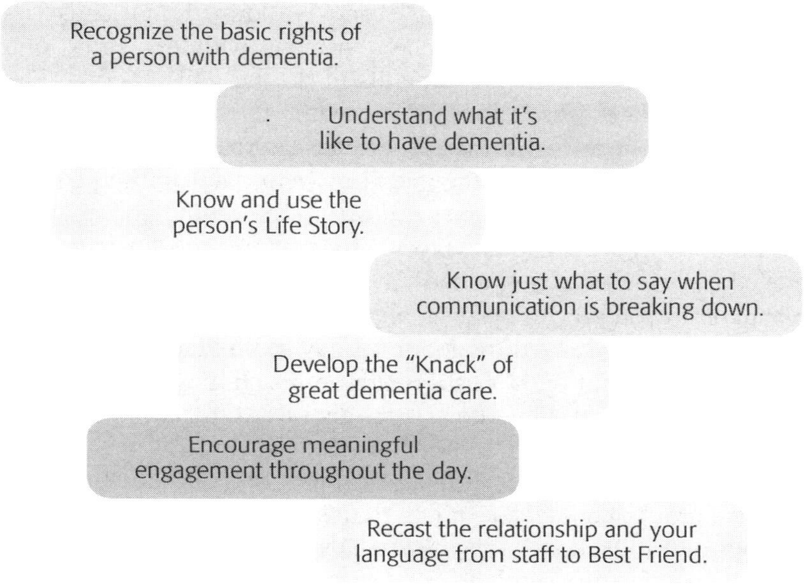

Recognize the basic rights of
a person with dementia.

Understand what it's
like to have dementia.

Know and use the
person's Life Story.

Know just what to say when
communication is breaking down.

Develop the "Knack" of
great dementia care.

Encourage meaningful
engagement throughout the day.

Recast the relationship and your
language from staff to Best Friend.

Figure 2.3. Building blocks of the Best Friends approach.

- Develop the "Knack" of great dementia care.
- Encourage meaningful engagement throughout the day.
- Recast the relationship and your language from staff to Best Friend.

Recognize the basic rights of a person with dementia. To be a Best Friend, a care partner must support the basic rights of a person with dementia. Embracing each tenet of the Dementia Bill of Rights helps us see and acknowledge the person beneath the cloak of dementia, a person who deserves our best care and support and who has the right to live with choice and dignity.

Understand what it's like to have dementia. Behaviors that seem strange or unreasonable become easier to interpret or accept when you understand that dementia affects the brain. None of us would expect a friend with a broken arm to play softball with us. We can *see* the cast and know that the injury is real. In contrast, we can't *see* a broken brain, so instead of acting from compassion, we might incorrectly conclude that "she is just pushing my buttons" or "he could do more if he tried harder."

Understanding what it's like to have dementia helps us develop empathy. Best Friends staff use empathy to become more accepting, patient, and compassionate in meeting the needs of the person.

Know and use the person's Life Story. We know our friends well, our close friends even better. When persons with dementia forget their past, it's up to their Best Friends to do the remembering. Most dementia programs have a form or procedure for collecting key social and personal history—what the Best Friends approach calls the person's Life Story. In dementia care, the Life Story helps us help the person to recall happy times and successes (a hole-in-one on the golf course or a community award). The Life Story also gives us tools for redirection when the person is having a bad day (asking a woman who loves to bake to teach you how to make an apple pie).

Using the Life Story throughout the day to build a caring relationship is a key element of the Best Friends approach. For example, a Best Friends staff member who knows a resident lived in Hawaii might ask the person to teach a group some simple Hawaiian words or schedule a movie about surfing. The staff member might also offer the traditional Hawaiian greeting of "Aloha" or talk to the resident about a recipe for a delicious pineapple upside-down cake. Doing simple things inspired by the person's Life Story can help a resident feel safe, secure, and valued. (See Chapter 3 for an in-depth look at the Life Story.)

Know just what to say when communication is breaking down. Dementia damages a person's ability to communicate. The person often has trouble making conversation, expressing his or her wishes verbally, and understanding requests. Making matters worse, the short-term forgetfulness that accompanies most types of dementia means that even if the person understands a question from you ("Barbara, can I help you brush your teeth?"), your words may soon be forgotten (the person says "Yes," but then walks out of the bathroom).

Friends talk a lot, text, e-mail, and even communicate with nonverbal language. The Best Friends staff member understands the importance of slowing down and being present for the person with dementia as well as using good communication skills. There is a wrong way and right way to communicate with a person with dementia, and the tips we share in Chapter 4 will help you build your skills.

Develop the "Knack" of great dementia care. Knack is the art of doing difficult things with ease or using clever tricks and strategies. How do we get the Knack? When we rethink or recast our relationship from staff member to Best Friend, our worldview changes. You practice patience and understanding. If the person says that she likes the current president, Bill Clinton, we don't correct her. Instead we might say, "I like him, too."

Knack is more fully developed and explained in Chapter 5. Much of it is intuitive, but other elements of Knack will be for you to think about and even practice. Almost everyone can learn elements of Knack, and once it's mastered can solve problems with greater finesse and experience more enjoyment, success, and satisfaction in being a care partner.

Encourage meaningful engagement throughout the day. Persons with dementia may no longer be able to take part in activities they once enjoyed or initiate new ones. Therefore, they can easily become isolated, bored, and frustrated. Prominent in the Best Friends approach is the idea that socialization is therapeutic; it can fight depression, keep people physically fit, and foster feelings of happiness and success.

Chapter 6 discusses how to revitalize and strengthen your formal activity program. We also discuss how to draw more attention to the unstructured, "in the moment" times that fill most of our days. For example, a great residential care program may have four or five excellent activities on the calendar *and* have staff who spend time together with a resident taking short walks, talking, giving hand massages, or doing simple chores. In a Best Friends program, we call this "activities done with engagement."

Recast the relationship from staff to Best Friend. As you learn and begin to use the Best Friends approach, we encourage you to use the language of friendship throughout the day. When a team meeting is called to discuss a resident's behavior, ask how the staff can be a "Best Friend" to that person. Rework job descriptions to emphasize the importance of relationships. When you are spending one-on-one time with a person, let him or her know that you appreciate their friendship. Using the phrase *Best Friends* and developing authentic relationships ultimately helps the person feel safe, secure, and valued. A Best Friends program changes the culture, reflecting a caring community where all benefit.

Here's an example of how simple (but rewarding) a Best Friends approach can be:

> David Troxel's mother, Dorothy, was diagnosed with Alzheimer's disease in 1999. After being cared for at home for 7 years, she moved into memory care at Carlton Senior Living in Sacramento, California. On most days, she was upbeat, but she had occasional bad days. When this happened, staff would offer her a cup of Earl Grey tea with milk. "My mother was Canadian, and her parents were British," says David. "Earl Grey tea with milk was her favorite and represented past traditions and rituals. When staff (with lots of Knack) offered her this drink, she felt known and appreciated, and her worry would change to contentment."

The Carlton Senior Living staff often thanked Dorothy for being their friend, and she thanked them for being her friend. Friendship proved to be comforting and connecting. "When she died at the community after almost 2 weeks in hospice, I was deeply moved by how her Best Friends care partners would take shifts sitting with her," says David. "In fact, one of her Carlton Senior Living Best Friends, Hafida, came in on her own time to sit with her, along with me, my father, and our family friend Myra when she died."

How Friendship Works in the Context of Dementia Care

If you are new to the field of dementia care, it might be confusing to think that an in-home client, day center participant, or resident can be a friend. Maybe you've been taught to address someone as Mrs. Smith instead of Anne. Maybe you are worried about boundaries. Why is it so important to think about the elements of friendship as you go to work every day with 40 people with dementia? The reason goes back to our earlier discussion about empathy. It's easy for someone with dementia to get lost in confusion and feel disconnected from the flow of life. Without our intervention, the person can become isolated. As a Best Friends care partner, you reach through the cloud of dementia to call someone by his or her name, make a joke, comment on a piece of jewelry, or give a hug, which tells the person that you care. As in any good friendship, when the person knows a caring friend is offering support, he or she feels better and more confident.

We understand that boundaries exist and you need to bring a professional manner to your work, but people with dementia need your partnership. They need the people around them in ways that people without dementia may not. As Virginia Bell has said, "Persons with dementia may be confused about a lot of things, but they know if you are in relationship with them." Excellent dementia care is based on that relationship.

Best Friends Know Each Other's History and Personality

Typically, people become friends because they have something in common, such as graduating from the same high school or college, or an enthusiasm for Saturday night bowling. As the friendship grows, they learn more about each other: their families, birthdays and birthplaces, cultural and religious traditions, hobbies, and special achievements. As much as we think we know about our friends, there are often surprises, such as an opera-loving friend who secretly has a passion for country music.

Friends also become good judges of each other's moods and personalities. For instance, a friend develops a sense of timing by knowing when it's okay to tease someone and how. Friends even begin to understand each other's problem-solving style by knowing when a word of advice is welcome and when it may be resented.

In dementia care, Best Friends care partners get to know the person's history and personality by

- becoming the person's memory
- being sensitive to the person's values and spiritual traditions
- being sensitive to the person's culture
- learning the person's personality, moods, and problem-solving style

The Best Friends Care Partner Becomes the Person's Memory

It's often difficult to learn biographical information from someone with dementia. He may have forgotten much of the past or simply be unable to recall the names of people, places, or things in his life. The Best Friends staff should learn as much as possible about the person in order to offer cues and reminders of his previous achievements.

> "California regulations state that we cannot admit a person to memory care without a doctor's report or a TB test—Plymouth Village puts Life Story information in the same category. Having a rich Life Story when the person moves in allows us to meet their personal preferences and deliver the best, relationship-based care." (Connie Garrett, Director of Resident Services, Plymouth Village, Redlands, CA)

A good Life Story can tell you important details related to work, family, and spiritual traditions, but it can also reveal small facts that can make or break the day. Perhaps the person loves spicy food (so we know to have hot sauce available) or likes to sleep in her socks (thus allowing us to hold up a fun pair of red socks and offer them to her as she prepares to retire for the evening). Make the Life Story a priority!

The Best Friends Care Partner Is
Sensitive to the Person's Values and Spiritual Traditions

Even late in the illness, the person often retains his or her religious or spiritual traditions. It's important to ask the person and his or her family about spiritual practices. Did the person participate in a faith community? Did he or she find a spiritual connection through other means?

Percell Smith, Jr., is a vice president of resident loyalty for CHE Trinity Senior Living Communities in Livonia, Michigan. He leads the implementation of Sanctuary™, a person-centered model that honors the sacredness of every soul. "As a faith-based organization, we seek to understand each resident's spirituality. Taking the time to share a favorite hymn or inspirational reading with one of our residents is a gift. These precious moments enable us to develop relationships and share meaningful experiences with persons living with dementia."

Creating sacred moments and honoring traditions is part of being a Best Friends care partner. For example, if a new resident belongs to the Baha'i faith, finding out more about Baha'i will help you identify spiritual readings, music, or other elements of Baha'ism that will keep the person connected to these important traditions. When someone does not have a religious heritage or set of beliefs, look for other elements of his or her spirituality, whether it comes to them through being with children, the arts, or being in nature. (For an extended discussion of spirituality, religion, and dementia, see Chapter 9, "Inner Passage: Spiritual Journeying and Religion," in our book *A Dignified Life*.)

The Best Friends Care Partner Is Sensitive to the Person's Culture

In care communities, the care partner and person with dementia often come from different cultures. We once visited a Chicago building where more than two dozen languages were spoken and people came from all sorts of cultures and educational backgrounds. We believe that the Best Friends approach can cross cultures, but we also know that there is more to culture than remembering favorite foods or special holidays. A Best Friends care partner needs to be sensitive to aspects of culture that might be more hidden. Does the person come from a culture in which direct eye contact is considered rude? How are elders treated in this culture? The Life Story and conversations with family members will help you uncover what you need to know about a person's culture.

Kusang Tobdhen, a care partner at The Grove at Piedmont Gardens in Oakland, has been practicing the Best Friends approach for more than 3 years. Kusang is from Tibet, and many traditions in the United States have been new for him. The Best Friends approach has taught him to be patient, smile a lot, have fun, and provide lots of kind words. The caring culture of a Best Friends program has also helped him feel that the workplace is a community, a family, and not just a place to work. At The Grove, staff, families, and residents have also enjoyed getting to know Kusang as a Best Friends staff member. Kusang has taught the group much about his Tibetan culture and has enjoyed learning about the cultural backgrounds of the diverse residents.

Elements of Friendship and Dementia Care

Friends know each other's history and personality.
In dementia care, a Best Friend:

Becomes the person's memory

Is sensitive to the person's traditions

Learns the person's personality, moods, and problem-solving style

Friends do things together.
In dementia care, a Best Friend:

Involves the person in daily activities and chores

Initiates activities

Ties activities into the person's past skills and interests

Encourages the person to enjoy the simpler things in life

Remembers to celebrate special occasions

Friends communicate.
In dementia care, a Best Friend:

Listens skillfully

Speaks skillfully

Asks questions skillfully

Speaks using body language

Gently encourages participation in conversations

Friends build self-esteem.
In dementia care, a Best Friend:

Gives compliments often

Carefully asks for advice or opinions

Always offers encouragement

Offers congratulations

Friends laugh often.
In dementia care, a Best Friend:

Tells jokes and funny stories

Takes advantage of spontaneous fun

Uses self-deprecating humor often

Continued

Friends are equals.
  In dementia care, a Best Friend:
    Does not talk down to the person
    Always works to protect the dignity of the person, to "save face"
    Does not assume a supervisory role
    Recognizes that learning is a two-way street

Friends work at the relationship.
  In dementia care, a Best Friend:
    Is not overly sensitive
    Does more than 50% of the work
    Builds a trusting relationship
    Shows affection often

The Best Friends Care Partner Learns the Person's Personality, Moods, and Problem-Solving Style

Personalities and problem-solving styles do sometimes change with the onset of dementia, but more often than not the person's underlying attitudes and styles remain intact. For example, a person who always coped well with adversity may bring some of this resiliency into dementia. A person who has always been a take-charge individual or held positions of authority may not take kindly to being told what to do.

> When Joan Jorgensen of Hillsboro, Oregon, was diagnosed with younger-onset Alzheimer's, her Type A personality and strong work ethic proved challenging for staff. They asked Joan to be in charge of straightening "crooked paintings" on the wall, often sending a staff member ahead of her to tilt the various prints and paintings hanging on the single nail. Joan made her rounds and felt a great sense of accomplishment after her daily chore.

Best Friends Do Things Together

Many friendships start with common interests and deepen as friends enjoy going to movies, taking walks, playing sports, taking a trip or vacation, working on a volunteer project, doing crafts, going shopping, or simply talking on the phone. Good friends find that simply renting a video or going to the grocery store together can give as much pleasure as an elaborately planned outing. Whether planned or spontaneous, doing things together opens up opportunities for engagement—time spent in meaningful conversation, shared feelings, laughter, and the growth that comes from shared experiences.

In dementia care, the Best Friends care partner finds ways to do things together by

- involving the person in daily life
- initiating activities
- tying events and activities into the person's past skills and interests
- encouraging the person to enjoy the simple things in life
- remembering to celebrate special occasions

The Best Friends Care Partner Involves the Person in Daily Life

A person with dementia and a Best Friend can do a project together, such as cleaning the kitchen. Even with limited skills, the person can often help with daily chores, such as drying the dishes or stacking the newspapers to recycle. The key is to get the person involved, to encourage him or her to be a part of life.

The Best Friends Care Partner Initiates Activities

People with dementia often lose their "start button"—their ability to initiate activities and contribute in a meaningful way. Knowing a person's Life Story, their likes, dislikes and routines, provides an opportunity for engagement. A Best Friend could say, for example, "I would like to take a walk. Come on, join me! It's great to exercise with you and I know how you like your daily walk." Best Friends need to be there to encourage involvement in daily events.

> Molly Carpenter, Caregiver Advocate at Home Instead, Inc., franchisor of the Home Instead Senior Care franchise network, says that she and her colleagues encourage Home Instead® homecare workers, called CAREGivers℠, to take advantage of the surrounding details they will likely find in a senior's home. "You can start a conversation and a meaningful activity by looking at the pictures on the wall, dusting off old sports trophies, or admiring a collection of ceramic rabbits. It's up to the CAREgiver to jump-start a great day and give the senior's day meaning."

The Best Friends Care Partner Ties
Activities into the Person's Past Skills and Interests

Because people have led such full, rich lives, the possibilities for linking activities to the past are unlimited. For example, a resident who worked in a bakery may enjoy baking bread or muffins. Someone fluent in

Spanish might enjoy teaching staff some basic Spanish words. A piano player may still be able to play some favorite old tunes.

> Virginia enjoyed being a Best Friend to Patricia Estill, a participant in the Best Friends™ Day Center in Lexington, Kentucky. Virginia worked one-on-one to help Patricia continue her long-held passion for painting beautiful folk art pictures of African American women in colorful clothes. This activity engaged Patricia throughout her journey with dementia.

The Best Friends Care Partner Encourages the Person to Enjoy the Simple Things in Life

Simple things can still be meaningful to persons with dementia. Just like the rest of us, they enjoy a short walk around a park, sitting on a bench and watching the world go by, brushing a friendly dog, or completing a simple chore. Many residential dementia care programs take a weekly field trip to a museum or place of interest. But sometimes the drive itself is the most enjoyable part of the experience.

> David recalls the good times he and his father had taking his mother, Dorothy, out for a drive. "We would drive through old neighborhoods, admire the gardens, read some of the signs aloud, listen to some 1940s music on the car radio, and end up at a drive-in. It was fun to eat a small cheeseburger or have an ice cream while sitting in the car."

The Best Friends Care Partner Remembers to Celebrate Special Occasions

The ritual of a birthday party, anniversary celebration, Veteran's Day parade, or other long-held traditions can bring back many positive memories. Special occasions can be celebrated throughout the year, making a big day out of a birthday or other family event. Birthdays are especially significant. It's okay to have a monthly party for everyone born in a given month, but be sure to give each person a special day on his or her birthday!

> Jason Delamarter, vice president of business development for Prestige Care in Vancouver, Washington, recalls that his mother put out a special red plate on his birthday with the words, "You are special today." Prestige uses this plate, manufactured by a German company called Waechtersbach (and available in many U.S. department stores or online), in its memory care program to celebrate residents' birthdays.

Best Friends Communicate

The best friendships often involve a lot of talking. Whether it's over the phone or at work in the company break room, friends love to swap stories, gossip, share ideas, and confide in one another. Friends are also there to listen to each other, in good and bad times.

In dementia care, Best Friends Care Partners communicate by

- listening carefully
- speaking skillfully
- asking questions thoughtfully
- using and paying attention to body language
- gently encouraging participation in conversations

The Best Friends Care Partner Listens Carefully

In dementia care, it's important to try to be there for the person when he wants to talk about his feelings. Persons with dementia should be given time to share their feelings or ideas. Sometimes patience is rewarded with an insight.

> Celeste Lynch, director of wellness at Moorings Park in Naples, Florida, tells a story about spending time with a resident with mild cognitive impairment. The resident was taking part in a support group and activity program for people with early cognitive challenges. The resident told Celeste that her confusion was like being in a boat with "oars up" (floating down the river with no control). Now that she was in the support group and was in a safe place to share her feelings, she told Celeste, "My oars are now back in the water. I now feel more in control of my life."

Communication can come from the heart as well as from the head. By listening carefully to a person, even when he or she cannot be readily understood, it's often possible to get a clear message when we least expect it.

The Best Friends Care Partner Speaks Skillfully

The person should be given every opportunity to understand what is being said. A Best Friend should use short, simple, direct sentences with descriptive language, such as, "Please hand me my red purse," instead of "Hand me that thing." Also, we must remember to speak clearly, slowly, and loudly if the person has a hearing impairment.

> Ruth Eveland, a Best Friends™ Day Center participant and a long-time "dog person," used to own a breed called keeshonds. When you join her to look through her favorite book of dog breeds, she loves a general conversation about dogs but feels really known when you ask her to get into specifics, such as the differences between small dogs and big dogs, naming specific breeds, and, of course, talking about the personality of her beloved keeshonds.

The Best Friends Care Partner Asks Questions Thoughtfully

A person may become easily frustrated if asked questions she does not know the answer to. Thoughtful or skillful questions are ones that don't just have a yes or no response ("Do you like to go on picnics?"). They are more open-ended, have no right or wrong answers, and encourage friendly conversation ("What do you like best about a picnic?"). Find tips for creating thoughtful questions in the sidebar "Thoughtful Questions."

> Dr. Amy D'Aprix, a prominent gerontologist based in Toronto, Canada, has developed a series of cards with open-ended questions to encourage conversation. The Caring Cards encourage reminiscence and conversation and include questions like, "What do you think contributes to a happy marriage?" or "What are some of the greatest adventures you experienced as an adult?" Staff members using her cards hear fun and surprising answers. If the person stumbles or if the question doesn't evoke an easy answer, staff members just move on to the next card or answer the question themselves!

The Best Friends Care Partner Uses and Pays Attention to Body Language

Because verbal skills are diminished, body language becomes very important in dementia care. A Best Friend should greet the person warmly, smile broadly, and hold out a hand. Almost always, the person will respond with a handshake. (The handshake still holds special meaning with older people who remember a time when everyone in polite company would shake hands.) A mutual handshake is the beginning of a bond and is a deep-rooted symbol that one is a friend, not a foe.

In dementia care, talking with the hands is encouraged. Gestures such as tapping the seat on a chair can help the person get the message

Thoughtful Questions

Thoughtful or skillful questions are open-ended, have no right and wrong answers, and encourage friendly conversation.

[Use your knowledge of the person's Life Story]: *"What did you enjoy the most about growing up in New York City?"*

[Encourage a conversation during an activity]: *"Why do you think the Mona Lisa is smiling?"*

[Start a friendly debate]: *"Do you think cats make better pets or dogs? Why?"*

[Ask for life advice]: *"How long do you think someone should date before getting married?"*

[Engage in mealtime discussions]: *"What makes a good meatloaf?"*

to sit down. Just as important is paying attention to the body language and facial expressions of the person, especially as vocabulary diminishes.

> Sheryl Sparks of Ferndale, Washington, has worked in memory care for many years and led dementia programs for regional companies. She often teaches staff the power of making a positive first impression. "If you are coming to work in a bad mood, persons with dementia will pick up on that tension, and your day will go from bad to worse." Sheryl notes that a big smile and enthusiasm lift everyone's spirits. "If you are involved in [activities of daily living], starting out with some positive energy also instills confidence and supports cooperation and success." As a former bartender, Sheryl believes that having a fun-spirited job where you learn people's names, provide a welcome greeting, and keep the party going has served her well in her career in dementia care.

The Best Friends Care Partner Gently Encourages Participation in Conversations

It's important to include the person in everyday conversation as much as possible.

> Tricia Horgan from Peabody, Massachusetts, is a divisional director of the Life Guidance® memory program for Atria Senior Living. "I like to think of myself as the queen of chit chat. I talk to the ladies about my outfit and their outfits, help them with their rosary beads, sing a short song, and ask some questions. With just a bit of effort, I can begin to create some energy and conversation. The residents need us to get the ball rolling . . . then the magic happens." Tricia can take almost anything in the room or any part of her outfit and start a fun-filled conversation.

Best Friends Build Self-Esteem

A good friendship brings out the best in each person with dementia and builds self-esteem. It involves a mutual support system of giving each other constructive criticism and feedback and, when the chips are down, giving unconditional support. Friends look at strengths more than weaknesses.

In dementia care, Best Friends care partners build self-esteem by

- giving compliments often
- asking for advice or opinions
- offering encouragement
- offering congratulations

The Best Friends Care Partner Gives Compliments Often

Telling a person "You look nice today" or "You really did a good job gardening" builds self-esteem. A compliment can also "disarm" someone who is having a bad day or bad moment by distracting the person, moving him or her away from the problem or concern. Compliments inevitably evoke a smile.

> Jim Cox is the executive director of the Cascades of the Sierra in Reno, Nevada. "I've been so blessed to be with residents with dementia through much of my career. I'm a guy with a big personality, so the residents always take notice of my arrival. I take a few minutes to make the rounds, give some gentle hugs, and offer lots of compliments. It's my feel-good moment of the day—and I hope a great moment for them, too!"

The Best Friends Care Partner Carefully Asks for Advice or Opinions

Another way to show a person that she is valued is by asking for her opinion. The question need not be about the national debt or foreign trade. Instead, a man could ask, "I didn't have a chance to look in the mirror today. Do you think my tie matches my shirt?" This could lead to a lengthy discussion about fabrics, textures, colors, changing widths of ties, and perhaps even a new wardrobe. Everyone likes to be asked for an opinion; it shows we are valued.

> Kathy Laurenhue is a writer and programming consultant who specializes in keeping an active brain. She often wears something to spark interest, such as an unusual scarf, and as a prop for starting a conversation. She might begin with a self-doubt ("I like the design in this scarf, but do you think it goes well with my dress?"). She notes that, "They do tell you their honest opinion and will be the first to let you know if your outfit isn't quite coming together!" Props like clothing are an opening for discussions in which people talk about their own preferences, opinions, and share advice. You can learn more about her work in the Suggested Resources.

The Best Friends Care Partner Always Offers Encouragement

Persons with dementia need as much encouragement as possible, which can take many forms. Sometimes it's valuable to encourage the person by reminding her of her value as a friend: "You add so much to my life" or "We're just like sisters." The person can also be encouraged to attempt a particular task, especially one that seems possible to accomplish. A Best Friend might say, "I could use your help in putting this puzzle together. Would you sit by me and help out?"

> Nancy Schier Anzelmo is a faculty member in the Gerontology Department at California State University, Sacramento, and the principal of Alzheimer's Care Associates. In her role as a consultant she supports many residents in residential care. She says that a key ingredient of successful programs is staff members who get the simple things right by, for example, sitting and being with a person with dementia and encouraging engagement. "Simple efforts can yield big results and make the day more interesting and fun for everyone."

The Best Friends Care Partner Offers Congratulations

In dementia care, the person should be congratulated often for small and big successes.

> Staff at the Best Friends™ Day Center knew that Pauline Huffman was the first woman in Lexington, Kentucky, to ever bowl a sanctioned perfect 300 game. For this accomplishment, she was inducted into the Lexington Bowling Association's Hall of Fame. She also once made a hole-in-one in golf. Pauline may not have understood or even recalled all of the details of her athletic accomplishments, but she knew something important had happened and loved being reminded of her past.

Best Friends Laugh Often

Humor helps people enjoy shared experiences, relieves tension, and brings people together. Many researchers have also confirmed that laughter has positive physiological effects, such as boosting the immune system and lowering blood pressure.

> Kathy Laurenhue, who is active in the Association for Applied and Therapeutic Humor, says "Laughter is an essential door opener to communication, and in tragedy it gives us momentary hope. It involves both having a good sense of humor—laughing easily—and being "in good humor,' meaning cheerful. It's tied to happiness, play, creativity, pleasure, and well-being. Cultivate it in everything you do."

In dementia care, Best Friends care partners help their friends laugh often by

- telling jokes and funny stories
- taking advantage of spontaneous fun
- using self-deprecating humor often

The Best Friends Care Partner Tells Jokes and Funny Stories

Even the corniest joke can evoke big laughs from someone with dementia. Funny stories are also popular, particularly ones that involve either the care partner or the person. For example, a Best Friends care partner might say, "I still haven't forgiven you for eating the last piece of pie." We should not forget that the person can sometimes remember or tell a great story or joke.

It can almost be a running joke in some friendships ("Not that story again, I've heard it before!"). Yet in dementia care, a story that is repeated often can be a favorite of the person. It may be that he or she simply cannot remember having heard it before. More likely, the person connects with the smiles, laughter, and joy associated with the story.

The Best Friends Care Partner Takes Advantage of Spontaneous Fun

Things happen spontaneously that are often humorous for a person with dementia and the people around him. Laughter can come from watching staff at a nursing community chase a pet rabbit that has gotten free from its cage.

> Tracy Byrne works at the Best Friends™ Day Center. "I don't always have a planned activity, but that's more than okay. I focus more on spontaneity. It's amazing how the day is full of surprises when I let go of my need for planning and just go with it!"

The Best Friends Care Partner Uses Self-Deprecating Humor Often

Friends are not afraid to be the butt of their own jokes. Embarrassing moments happen to all of us but are a particular concern of people with dementia. When a person forgets a name of an old friend, a good response from a Best Friend could be "That's okay, I'm glad I'm not the only one who forgets things" or "I looked all over for my glasses last week and then found them—right on my nose." What self-deprecating humor does is reassure the person that she is not the only one in the world who can be forgetful. It also defuses negative situations and helps the person stay in a positive mood. A good self-deprecating remark also allows for laughter to break the tension, for a frown to turn into a smile.

> Best Friends Expert Trainer Tonya Cox often jokes about a wardrobe malfunction or mistake, or the latest adventure she had with her children. Residents at Homeplace at Midway and Christian Care Communities where she works enjoy her stories because they can relate. The stories also reassure participants that they're not the only ones who make mistakes.

Best Friends Are Equals

No friendship will survive condescending behavior. Everyone has different strengths and weaknesses, but differences should be celebrated rather than dwelled on. The Best Friends™ Dementia Bill of Rights (see Chapter 1) reminds us that persons with dementia have the right to be treated as adults, to be listened to, and to be afforded respect for their feelings and point of view.

In dementia care, Best Friends care partners nurture respect and equality by

- not talking down to the person
- always working to protect the person's dignity and save face
- not assuming a supervisory role
- recognizing that learning is a two-way street

How to Become a Best Friends Care Partner

How can you begin to apply the Best Friends approach in your work? Here are some perspectives about the approach that we've assembled from staff who are practicing the approach in a variety of settings. Which statements seem most meaningful or important to you? What would you add to the list?

Recognize the basic rights of a person with dementia

I will be an advocate for the person to get the best care and support. I will treat the person like I'd want to be treated. I will encourage my team members to listen and show respect. I'll try my best to include her as part of our community and world. She could be my mom—let's all treat her like our mom.

Understand what it's like to have dementia

I will walk a mile in his shoes to understand that dementia can be a frightening and frustrating experience. I'll be more understanding when he's having a bad day. I won't take things personally. I'll be there for him on good and bad days. I'll learn as much as I can about dementia. Thinking about his experience helps me develop patience and empathy.

Know and use the person's Life Story

I will learn all I can about each person I care for. I will talk to him about his interesting life in the military. I'll ask her about all the cool things in her apartment. Each resident must have a great story. I will find out her favorite foods and ask her for recipes. I'll ask her to teach me some words in French. She likes to teach me about how to be a good hostess—how to set a table and host a good dinner party. Let's also try to learn more about each other as team members.

Know just what to say when communication is breaking down

I'll come to work with smiles instead of frowns. I'll ask the resident who was a head nurse for advice about my options for a nursing career. Give lots of compliments. Use positive body language. Offer her some simple choices to help her feel I respect her. I'll slow down and speak up. I'll listen more carefully. It's fun when you finally get on the same track. I feel we communicate well.

Develop "the Knack" of great dementia care

I love the Knack idea—I think I have it. Not everyone has the Knack, but we can all learn. The hardest one is patience. Knack is all about loving the residents. Knack to me is telling him I'm his friend and then seeing him smile and tell me that he is my friend. Staff who can't get the Knack should work somewhere else. I love the idea that it only takes 30 seconds to use the Knack.

Continued

Help the person stay engaged throughout the day

Boredom is the enemy. I want to bring my own interests to the day center program. Keep things more adult. I think they do so much better when it's a full and busy day. I'll do my best to use the outdoor space more. The activity calendar is just the beginning. . . . It's also important to do short, in-the-moment things. Music is magic. I like to exercise, so why not do it with the residents? I think one reason they love the day program is that it gives them so many things to do.

Recast the relationship from staff to Best Friend

Best Friends is a new way of doing my job. My company rewrote our job descriptions, and we all had to sign up to be a Best Friend—kind of cool to be paid to be a friend! I'm convinced that relationships help everyone feel better and do better. My nursing home has been kind of a depressing place to work. With Best Friends we are getting our enthusiasm and energy back. Everyone needs a Best Friend, particularly our residents with dementia.

The Best Friends Care Partner Does Not Talk Down to the Person

Condescending language is never appropriate in good dementia care. Examples of inappropriate language include speaking in an exaggerated, slow, and measured voice when unnecessary; being insensitive; using childlike language; being flippant; not giving the person time to respond to a question; asking inappropriate and embarrassing questions; or "talking through" a person as though he or she were not present.

> Tonya Cox regularly visits the memory care neighborhoods and day centers operated by Christian Care Communities. "Treating our day center participants and residents with dignity and respect are core values for our organization. I always model this to our team members, greeting the person by his or her preferred name, using adult language and a normal tone of voice, giving choices and treating the person as an adult. I think this ongoing modeling is even more important than what you discuss in a training program."

The Best Friends Care Partner Always Works to Protect the Dignity of the Person, to "Save Face"

Many persons with dementia remain fiercely proud. A good example of "saving face" is letting the person off the hook if she fails. If someone asks an awkward question ("How many children do you have?") and a Best Friend can see the person struggling, she can jump in and provide an answer, change the subject, or tell a self-deprecating joke so that the person will not feel humiliated.

When Margaret Brubaker's friends or family visited, they were often concerned that she was not eating well. She was very proud and refused gifts of food, saying that she was not hungry or had "just eaten an enormous meal!" A volunteer took a different approach. During one visit, he said, "Margaret, you could do me such a favor. Bananas were on sale this week and I bought 3 pounds. My wife went to the store separately and she bought 3 pounds. We just don't know what to do with all these bananas. It would help us so much if you'd take some off our hands." Margaret took the bananas with delight because she was doing her friend a favor.

The Best Friends Care Partner Does Not Assume a Supervisory Role

Good friendships usually don't involve being bossed around, and the person often responds negatively to feeling controlled. Offering simple choices is one way to help persons with dementia feel they are respected and have a voice in their daily lives.

Plaza Assisted Living in Honolulu, Hawaii, calls its memory care program Hali'a (roughly translated from the Hawaiian as "celebrating cherished memories"). The company embraces the Best Friends philosophy in its program, which teaches staff to offer simple choices to residents. Tricia Medeiros, Chief Operating Officer and Best Friends Master Trainer, supports the importance of choice: "I want our residents to be the boss, not us. We encourage them to be part of the plan for the day, vote on movies to watch or places to go. We may have a word game planned, but our engagement staff can rearrange the day if our residents want to enjoy some outdoor time on one of our often spectacular days in Hawaii."

The Best Friends Care Partner Recognizes that Learning Is a Two-Way Street

Equality means learning things from each other. Many volunteers who work in adult day centers or long-term care communities comment that they learn much from the people they care about. Many persons with dementia can still share stories from their personal histories, express compassion and concern, or demonstrate old skills and hobbies.

Dicy Jenkins was a walking encyclopedia of information about plants and herbs used for health and healing. She knew how to use juniper berries, ginseng, feverfew, bee pollen, and burdock root for medicinal purposes. Volunteers at the adult day center often took copious notes on Dicy's remedies to relieve their ailments.

Best Friends Work at the Relationship

Every friendship has its difficult moments. Something said is misconstrued, or a friend disappoints. Clearly no friendship will survive a continuing series of disappointments, but friends discuss disagreements and work them out. It sometimes takes work to be a good friend, but the payoff is great.

In dementia care, Best Friends care partners work at the relationship by

- not being overly sensitive
- building trust
- showing affection often

The Best Friends Care Partner Is Not Overly Sensitive

Best Friends must recognize that challenging behaviors, when they occur, are normally part of the disease process, not part of the person. Sometimes, inhibitions are reduced by dementia. The person may say some surprising things.

> Geri Greenway valued great art, music, stylish clothes, and beautiful jewelry. When a volunteer in the day center program asked Geri what she thought of some new costume jewelry she had brought to the day program to display, Geri replied, "Well, it looks like a bunch of junk to me." The experience of the volunteer showed when she laughed and told the group, "Ask a question, get an answer."

The Best Friends Care Partner Builds Trust

Trust can become an issue with persons with dementia when they are uncertain about their surroundings or suspicious of their care partners. The person may not understand why they cannot drive any more or why they are at the day center. Trust is built into friendship through emotional connection, communication, and honesty.

> Helen King was very distrustful of the concept of an adult day center when she first attended one. She was very aware of her memory loss and did not want to expose her limitations. As she became familiar with the program volunteers, she realized that they were very supportive and respectful of her remaining abilities. Gradually, her trust grew, and she spoke enthusiastically about attending her "class" each day. Staff found that a calm, consistent approach helped Helen feel comfortable. They focused on taking her concerns seriously, answering her questions, and providing support. Helen became one of the great success stories, truly loving the program.

The Best Friends Care Partner Shows Affection Often

Some long-term care communities and adult day centers have a "three hugs a day" rule. Best Friends show the person with dementia affection as often as possible, through compliments, holding hands, a pat on the back, smiles, and hugs (why not three hugs an hour?). The Best Friends™ Day Center practices all kinds of hugs: group hugs, bear hugs, one-on-one hugs, and new ones invented in the spur of the moment.

> Tom Alaimo, Vice President of Memory Care Operations (Life Guidance®) for Atria Senior Living, has a gratifying job supporting more than 100 memory care neighborhoods and leading a team of dementia specialists in the field. "In addition to providing quality care and facilitating a healthy program of activities and engagement, we remain focused on compliance to meet Atria's high-quality standards, which in many cases exceed state regulations. I like to remind every employee in our company that our primary role is to show affection, kindness, and warmth toward our seniors with memory impairments so they know how much we truly care for them."

Conclusion

Who is your best or close friend? Your brother or sister? Your daughter? A college buddy? Your spouse or partner? Why are they your best friend? Recently, a group shared with us the qualities of their best friends. Being loyal and trustworthy, a good listener, someone who accepts me at my best and worst and knows me well, someone who makes me laugh and brings out the best in me—doesn't it sound familiar? We hope you'll agree with us that these are the very same qualities of a Best Friends staff.

PART 2

Best Friends in Your Care Setting

Now that you have mastered the basic principles of the Best Friends™ approach, you are ready to begin bringing the philosophy to life in your day-to-day work.

This section outlines how to create a therapeutic environment in your care setting using the Best Friends approach. A therapeutic environment starts with real knowledge of the person with dementia: his or her history, preferences, and pastimes. Also key is communicating with the person in ways that affirm and respect despite decreasing language and cognitive abilities. Activities large and small, planned and spontaneous can keep the person grounded in essential relationships and engaged with the world around him or her. Not every moment will go well, but you can be prepared to help the person achieve the best possible quality of life.

This section ends with a discussion of behavior, an important topic for anyone working in dementia care. Is there a way to turn a challenge into a success? We believe the answer is yes. A well-informed Best Friends care partner can solve problems and bring creative ideas to many common behavioral challenges.

Let's start with the Life Story—an essential element of good dementia care and the difference between success and failure as a care partner.

CHAPTER 3

The Life Story

How well do you know your friends? Even if they are just casual friends, we can usually name their occupations, marital status, general interests, favorite foods, type of car, hobbies, and other details. Social media adds to the picture, with regular updates from Facebook or Twitter or shared projects on Pinterest.

What about our *closest* friends? We know much more about them, including family history and traditions, likes and dislikes, even some of their secrets! We also know their strengths and weaknesses and understand their basic personalities. We know how to cheer them up when they are having a bad day, when to give advice (or not), and how to turn a *no* into a *yes*.

How do we learn so much about our friends? We get to know them by doing things together (hiking, working in the same office, going out to eat). We talk with each other (a date gone wrong, the stock market, or favorite bands or television shows). We share common interests (sports, binge watching a television series on Netflix, love of travel, or fitness and exercise).

As we get to know one another, these details are revealed gradually. But often a person with dementia can't share his or her own story, and as care partners in busy and complex long-term care settings, we don't have the luxury to learn a person's Life Story over time. To be an effective Best Friend, we need to know as much as we can on the first day of our relationship with the person and regularly add to our store of information, which must be collected and then incorporated into daily situations.

You've seen the power of the Life Story in our relationship with Rebecca Riley. The fact that we knew so much about her gave us almost endless tools and approaches to bring up favored subjects, reminisce, and help her achieve the best possible quality of life.

Rebecca taught us that the Life Story can be the difference between success and failure as a care partner. Because it's an essential element of great dementia care, it's a key principle in our Dementia Bill of Rights. It's a person's right to be known and be among people who care. To help ensure that right, we need to learn a lot about the person and incorporate that into our everyday relationship.

Knowing a lot about the person deepens and enriches the care partner relationship. You can use this knowledge to bring up favorite memories and special achievements, provide cues, and take advantage of past preferences and interests. Life Story information enhances conversation, helps customize activities, allows us to better understand behavior, and helps us redirect with greater success.

Since we championed the importance of the Life Story in our first edition of this book, collecting social and biographical history has become pretty universal in dementia care programs. But as we have traveled throughout the United States and even internationally, we've learned that this seemingly easy element of dementia care remains elusive. Here are some of the barriers we've seen:

- marketing staff who get all of the financial and medical forms completed but then say to the family, "Here is the Life Story questionnaire . . . please get it back to us when you can."
- Life Story information that is hidden away in charts or electronic records and not easily accessible to staff
- incomplete forms
- forms that are rarely updated with changing events, such as a new grandchild
- lack of training on what to do with the Life Story information once you have it

Even in programs that are doing a good job, staff routinely tell us that they wish they knew more or that there is no ongoing effort to remind staff about the importance of the Life Story focus. William "Billy" Small, Jr., owner of the Fountainview Center, a dementia community in Atlanta, Georgia, noticed that his staff, despite all of their efforts, would read residents' obituaries and say, "I never knew that!" This was Billy's wake-up call to double down on emphasizing the importance of the Life Story with his staff. "We should never be surprised by an obituary; we should know their life stories well."

Preparing the Life Story

The first step in preparing the Life Story is to collect the information. The staff member who collects information is often the first to meet with the person with dementia or family members (usually a sales or marketing team member or program coordinator). In skilled nursing, a social worker or nurse may bring his or her expertise to the process.

To collect information, consider making a visit to the new resident's home, if possible. A grand piano, a shelf of sports trophies, a library of travel books, an easel and art supplies, a kitchen gleaming with copper kettles and cookbooks—these are all revealing details. Start with the person; even with dementia, he or she may be able to recount a lot about his or her life. Then talk with family and friends. Remind all involved that this information is vital for your efforts to help the person transition into the program.

Get as much of the Life Story questionnaire filled out as possible beforehand, and then develop a process to add to the form in the first few weeks as staff get to know the person. The person will often express personal preferences around food, attend some activities more than others, or demonstrate routines that staff should know (reading a newspaper in the morning or watching late-night television).

If you are in a setting where time is of the essence and no Life Story is on hand—for example, working in an emergency room or driving an ambulance—it can be helpful to ask the person or the responsible party for a few quick insights ("He likes to be called Major Mike" or "She loves her cats"). Addressing someone by a preferred name or talking about those cats may calm the person, ease fears, and help a physician or EMT perform needed procedures without struggle.

Ingredients of the Life Story

The Recipe for the Life Story in Figure 3.1 outlines the ingredients of a comprehensive written Life Story of someone with dementia. Keep in mind that just as recipes differ, so do Life Stories. We can choose the important information to include in the Life Story that we write. But let's not create too bland a meal; we want to spice it up with interesting stories and fun facts about the person.

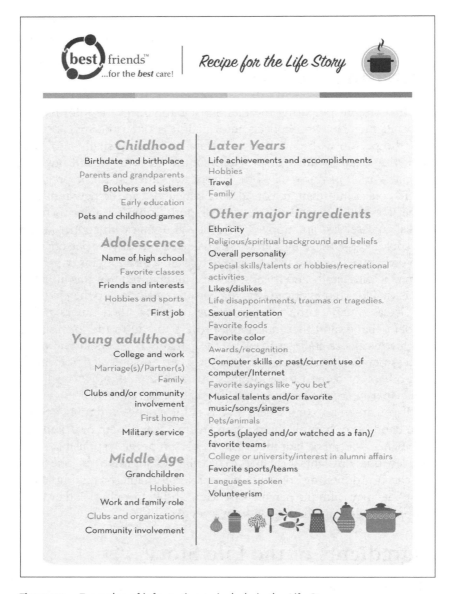

Figure 3.1. Examples of information to include in the Life Story.

Childhood

In dementia care, understanding the person's earliest years is sometimes more important than familiarity with the later years. Even well into their dementia, many people recall their childhoods. We want to know as much as possible about this influential time.

Although birthdate and place are a good place to start, we want to do more than simply record the basics. We want to get a feel for the environment in which the person was raised. Was the birthplace rural or urban? Was the person raised in a small town or big city? What were the town's main industries? Did the town have any special claim to fame? Someone might remember his or her hometown as the birthplace of the computer, where Coca-Cola was first bottled, or where everyone considered the Eiffel Tower the city's center. Velma Beaty enjoys being teased about the unusual name of her birthplace, Kissing Ridge, Kentucky. An old friend who lives in Stockbridge, Massachusetts, notes with pride that it's the hometown of the famed American painter and illustrator Norman Rockwell and that members of her family appear in his paintings. When available, this information can be a fascinating part of the Life Story.

Even a simple family tree of the person's childhood, with the names of his or her grandparents, parents, and siblings, can be important. Find out whether there were any particularly influential relatives, such as an adored older sister or a grandmother who baked prize-winning apple pies. Learn as much as possible about these key relatives. At one adult day center, staff were amazed to learn that 3 of the 15 participants in that day's program had a twin. At a residential community, a woman in memory care loved to talk about being the only girl in a large family of boys. She proudly called herself a "tomboy" and loved to talk about running around barefoot.

Does the person remember his or her first day of school? This is usually a milestone. Was school enjoyable? Was the person a good student? Was there a favorite subject or favorite teacher? We remember one woman who took pride in remembering that she was "Miss Seventh-Grade Square Root," and she enjoyed the laughter and words of congratulation that followed when she mentioned it!

Be sure to discover the occupation of the person's parents. Many people with dementia can recall their father's medical practice or mother's teaching career (or perhaps something not as typical for that era—maybe the mother flew a plane!).

Many older people emigrated or were children or grandchildren of immigrants. It's often meaningful to find out the country from which the family emigrated and how the family found its way to the United States. Sometimes these stories involve high drama, such as a life-threatening escape from a dangerous or oppressed country.

Discussing family roots is an excellent opportunity to ask questions about cultural traditions, especially if the person is an immigrant. What should care partners know about the culture, how it treats elders, its view on the family, and its beliefs about dress and personal expression?

Also inquire about life-defining childhood events. We certainly hope to find happy childhood experiences, but we want to understand any traumas in order to avoid triggering unhappy memories. It can be valuable to know whether a person had a troubled childhood (e.g., parents divorcing at an early age, surviving a wartime childhood). Also important are childhood traumas (perhaps the death of a close friend or a natural disaster such as a flood or fire).

A defining moment might be having been elected student body president or winning a statewide academic contest. Or maybe it was the day the person's father was elected to the state legislature. It can be valuable to get a feel for major geographic moves during childhood. If someone was a "military brat," for example, and lived in many towns and cities, this can be of interest. Family names are also important and are an ongoing source of conversation and comment.

"I loved my father. His name was Tobe. I named our daughter, Toby, for him," Willa McCabe explained proudly.

Henrietta Frazier enjoys sharing the story about her name. "My father died before I was born, so my mother named me Henrietta, for my father. His name was Henry."

We can also comment on the many interesting names from the past: "Your father's name was Zachariah and your mother's name was America—isn't that interesting!" Although they are sometimes dreaded and disdained, nicknames are important to record. Also of note are affectionate names for parents: Mama, Mother, Ma, Pa, Daddy, or Father.

Try to uncover favorite activities, hobbies, and games from childhood. Sports like hockey, softball, and football may have played a large role. Playground games can be recalled and even reenacted. More serious recreational activities, such as playing a musical instrument or collecting stamps and coins, can also be part of a comprehensive Life Story.

Researching Hometowns Online

The Internet can be a rich source of information and inspiration about early childhood locales. A quick search related to a childhood in New Orleans might reveal a picture of the person's house (Google Earth), or traditions such as Mardi Gras, local Cajun dishes, jazz music, or famous sites such as Bourbon Street (YouTube or Wikipedia).

Many of us retain vivid and pleasurable memories of childhood pets. Was there a special cat or dog in the person's childhood, perhaps a black cat named Midnight, a collie just like Lassie, or a pet deer on an Idaho ranch? People who grew up in rural areas might recall winning a ribbon for a prize animal at a state fair, or a pig that the family loved too much to eat.

Adolescence

Adolescence is one of the most influential life stages. Key life events during this time can include graduating from junior and senior high

When Memories Are Unhappy

Researchers suggest that humans are wired to remember happy rather than unhappy memories. One exception seems to be trauma, which can affect a person's life for many years. Although a Best Friends team will naturally focus on positive memories and try to evoke happy times for the people we serve, we will encounter some who have survived traumatic experiences, from the Holocaust and other war-related events to childhood trauma, abusive relationships, losing a parent or child, or even a single incident, such as being bitten by a dog.

Note these experiences as you collect Life Story material and attend to them. Knowing that someone is afraid of dogs or had a difficult time helps staff avoid sensitive topics or deal with them in a meaningful way when they arise. If someone recounts a troubled relationship with a parent, staff can listen with empathy, to let the person know that he or she is now valued and loved, and then try to redirect.

school, dating, and getting a first car and first job. Adolescence is also a time when children gain greater independence from parents—the first steps to adulthood.

Education is often a good starting point when covering this part of a Life Story. It's always good to know what kind of educational experience the person had. Did he or she complete high school? For many older adults, educational opportunities weren't a given. Many of them might have been the first in their family to graduate from college, often a source of great pride.

What other life events were associated with school? Many people might have had successful school experiences, such as being on the football team or cheerleading squad, or winning the local spelling bee. Experiences such as high school proms are memorable and often are photographed for scrapbooks, which can be retrieved and used as part of the Life Story.

Obtaining a driver's license can be a milestone. What was the person's first car? One California day center director told us that a discussion of "my first car" was one of the center's most successful programs. Even participants with poor memory seemed to be able to recall the make and color of their first car and that car's first flat tire.

Jobs are often the most important way people define themselves. A complete Life Story should discuss the person's first job. It can be interesting to ask about the person's first wage. Many young people would certainly be surprised to hear that the minimum wage in some states in 1974 was $2 an hour!

Perhaps a fitting way to end the written Life Story of this exuberant period is to ask the person if he or she can remember his or her first kiss. This question almost always evokes a laugh or a smile.

Young Adulthood

Education, work, and family life often dominate the young adult years. Of course we want to obtain information about whether the person married and whether he or she has children. Write down notes about his or her spouse: name, occupation, and, if available, some favorite stories from the marriage (e.g., their first home, their first trip to Europe). Most people enjoy talking about their children, so we want to know their names, where they live, occupations, and more. If the person remained single, we might find out more about any siblings with whom he or she remained close, and whether there were nieces or nephews or special cousins who made up his or her extended family.

Many people seek higher education during this period or begin working. A good Life Story incorporates the person's higher education (if any) and describes early work or career choices.

A wedding can be a highlight of this time of life, and a Life Story should include information about the wedding ceremony, especially any funny stories that can be recounted, such as the groom misplacing the ring or a multilevel cake that collapsed. Wedding pictures, part of most family's archives, can be a marvelous source of family history.

We should obtain as much information as we can about the person's job or career. Was he or she a doctor, farmer, house painter, homemaker, electrician, or artist? Any collections or materials from the person's work that might still be available can be noted. An architect might still have his or her drawings. A homemaker might have kept an elaborate card file of recipes. We can make note of whether the person wore special clothing associated with his or her occupation, such as a military or nurse's uniform, chef's apron, or farmer's overalls.

Some products might have a corporate logo that is meaningful to the person. He or she might very much enjoy wearing an old workplace cap or looking at letterhead with a company logo. Sometimes employee personnel manuals, military discharge papers, diplomas, licenses, or other documents can be found that are important artifacts of a person's career.

Often, this period is one in which the person purchased his or her first home, an act that has enormous symbolic value. When possible, pictures of the first house should be included in the Life Story. A surprising number of persons with dementia may still remember the amount of their first monthly mortgage payment. We can find out how many bedrooms the house had, what it looked like, and whether it had land surrounding it or was located on a small city lot.

Middle Age

Writing a complete Life Story of a person's middle-age period could fill several books, but again we want to highlight major themes to better understand his or her past. Middle age is a period in life when a person typically reaches the peak of his or her career. What was his or her last job before retirement, and was there any noteworthy achievement? It can be important to understand whether the person's identity is tied to his or her job. Some people identify themselves first and foremost as a doctor, engineer, plumber, or farmer. For others, job and work were secondary to their identity as father, wife, brother, or stepmother.

Avocations often develop during this time. We should find out what hobbies the person had or what recreational activities he or she enjoyed. Golfers often have spent countless hours thinking, talking, and sometimes anguishing over their game. If the person was a golfer (or still golfs), did he or she ever hit a hole in one? Was the person a champion bridge player? Did the person regularly use a computer and Internet?

We should also find out what happened during this time to the person's family. Did children marry? Were there grandchildren? Annual family reunions?

Later Years

For many people, retirement provides a chance to pursue a hobby or activity more avidly; the person who played bridge only once a month can now play three times a week. Another can go salmon fishing every week during the season. For many people, gardening is a pleasurable activity, and the Life Story should note favorite flowers and whether the person had special success with vegetables. Perhaps one year there was an 80-pound pumpkin in the garden!

Did the person have an active retirement period? Former President Jimmy Carter's mother, Miss Lillian, joined the Peace Corps to engage in meaningful volunteer work at age 68. What a mistake it would have been for a biographer to leave out this fact when describing her life!

Did the person remain physically active? Some older adults work out at health clubs, bike across the country, or take weekly organized hiking trips. If he or she decided to spend the retirement years sitting on the front porch watching the world go by, a note can be made to tease about the rocking chair that occupied his or her day.

Retirement is often a time for travel, and a special vacation can still be a vivid memory even for a person with dementia. Was there one "trip of a lifetime" or yearly vacation spot? What was the special attraction: a tropical island or a desert hideaway? Are pictures or souvenirs available that can be used for the Life Story?

Many retired people volunteer in their communities. Find out whether the person volunteered in a hospital auxiliary, for a local non-profit organization, or for a church or youth group. Noting someone's contributions to the community in a Life Story can be very valuable.

For example, a day center might even take a field trip to tour the library building named after a participant.

Some retired people use this period to enrich their lives through continuing education, formal or informal. Find out whether the person was an avid reader, learned any new skills during this time, or developed a new business.

Other Major Ingredients

Certainly an important part of any Life Story is the person's cultural, religious, and ethnic background and what role this background played throughout his or her life. Is the person Jewish, and did he or she keep kosher and attend synagogue or temple? Were there family traditions celebrating the person's African American heritage? Conversely, it's also important to note if someone has no strong religious background. Perhaps he or she would feel uncomfortable singing gospel songs at the residential care community.

It's also important to be aware of sexual orientation. In the past, many older adults would hide their identities if they were gay or lesbian. Today, growing awareness and acceptance is such that many people disclose their sexual preferences, and gay-friendly senior housing is becoming common in large cities. We want to capture this important information, train staff on diversity issues, and be welcoming to the person's partner or same-sex spouse.

One often-overlooked part of a Life Story is a person's awards or major achievements. Winning a prize or award is such a major event that it remains in the memory longer than many other events. Was the person honored with a Silver Star during Vietnam or with an award for Volunteer of the Year or Teacher of the Year?

In writing the Life story, it's also valuable to ask the person or his or her family additional questions. Did he or she have any strong likes or dislikes? At a day center group, one participant answered that question by saying "Republicans," and another in the same group replied "Democrats." We tried to steer clear of politics that day.

Some people have their own special "trademark" phrases, such as "You bet!" or "Two heads are better than one," that can add flavor to the person's Life Story. Ever since Best Friends™ Day Center participant Joan Wyzenbeek performed off-Broadway in the play *Gypsy*, she has loved the line from the play, "Bump it with the trumpet." When Joan seems worried or upset, Assistant Director Tracy Byrne smiles, makes eye contact, and just begins saying this funny phrase slowly and clearly. Joan catches on right away and says "Bump it with the trumpet" with enthusiasm and joy that can last for hours. It's a great example of Virginia Bell's observation that one happy moment can last the whole day.

An important part of the Life Story is the kinds of food the person enjoyed or enjoys. Many people spend a lot of time thinking about food. Some pride themselves on knowing special recipes or how to cook foods that reflect their ethnicity. Food can still be a source of much enjoyment and sensory pleasure for the person.

We also should know a person's favorite song or type of music. It's important to let people listen to music they enjoy, be it Bach, Benny Goodman, or the Beatles.

Although it seems unimportant, we should find out the person's favorite color. Often, late into dementia a person can still respond to questions about color and is pleased to be surrounded by items or wear clothing of a favored color.

Sports play a big role, particularly for people who follow—or even played—a variety of college and professional sports. Note in the Life Story any special fan loyalties or favorite sports.

The Life Story should also include special skills. For example, often a person will retain the ability to play a beautiful old song that he or she has played for many years, despite the fact that dementia makes learning a simple new song impossible. Other common skills include cooking, sewing, painting, and making crafts.

Unconventional questions, such as the ones shown in the "Questions that Enrich a Life Story" sidebar, can add extra richness to the Life Story. For example, a day center director writing a Life Story might ask the family whether the person might have held on to the first dollar earned or spent it the minute it came in. Maybe you will learn that your in-home client was a spender and loves to go to Macy's, so you can plan an occasional "shopping expedition."

The Life Story should take special note of any successes or happy memories that can be used to benefit the person. It should also offer warnings against any painful subjects, phobias, or important information to be avoided, if possible.

Harder to determine, but also of importance, is the overall personality of the person before he or she developed dementia. Learning this information is important because old personality patterns often are retained. Was he or she generally optimistic or pessimistic? What was his or her problem-solving approach? How did he or she handle stress?

Inevitably there will be gaps in the Life Story because family members may not be available to answer questions, or the person may not be able to share many details. If this is the case, we must do the best we can. No matter how many holes or mysteries, we are sure to make some discoveries as we go along.

Some gaps may be a result of progressing dementia. A devoted mother may eventually deny that she ever had a daughter, or a globetrotter may insist that he never traveled to Europe. In these cases, it's fine to gently cue the person, but sometimes we have to take note that this is not a topic to bring up or emphasize.

Preparing the Life Story gives us the foundation to touch distant memories, respect present preferences, and make a caring connection. Let's now see how we can best use this rich social history to deliver excellent care.

Questions that Enrich a Life Story

Play detective when writing a Life Story! Looking beneath the surface can pay many dividends in knowing the person with dementia better. Unusual questions can reveal much about the person's attitudes toward life, whether you learn the answers from the person or from friends and family. Because we are hoping to get an idea of the person's values before the onset of dementia, these questions are written in the past tense, but whenever possible, try to obtain present-day answers as well.

- How would the person have enjoyed spending New Year's Eve? In the middle of Times Square, out dancing, or home with a book?

- Did the person have a favorite book? Would he or she have preferred a good mystery novel, Shakespeare, the Bible, poetry, an auto repair manual, or The Old Farmer's Almanac?

- If the person was stuck on a desert island, what three things would he or she wish to have? (Assume that there is food, drink, and shelter.)

- How would the person's desk (or kitchen shelves and drawers, toolbox, or barn) have been organized?

- Would the person have looked at life thinking the glass is half full (optimist) or half empty (pessimist)?

- Would the person have held onto the first dollar he or she made or spent it right away?

Does It All Have to Be True?

Often, a person believes things about his or her life that are not factually correct. We strongly believe that they should be written into the story anyway and used.

Once, in the Best Friends™ Day Center program, Judge Jean Auxier signed his name "Senator Jean Auxier." Staff members asked his wife whether he had ever been a Kentucky state senator, thinking they had missed an important achievement in his written Life Story. Surprised, his wife said no, but he had always wanted to be! Although staff usually called Jean by his formal title, "Judge," now and then they slipped in "Senator." This pleased him very much. He won the "election" without ever campaigning!

Dicy Jenkins, another day center participant, claimed to have been born on a stagecoach in the Oklahoma territories, where she regularly spent time with an "Indian chief." Although her granddaughter said this wasn't true, when staff at the center asked Dicy about her time in Oklahoma, she would respond with rich stories, including one about a flirtatious chief having given her a turquoise ring. Upon hearing how handsome the chief was, one volunteer even joked, "Do you think he has a brother?"

Why not get into the person's reality and celebrate this part of his or her imagination? And who knows? Maybe the granddaughter was wrong!

How to Use the Life Story

All of the elements of the Life Story provide important tools for improving communication, making activities meaningful, preventing behaviors that are challenging to staff, and adding more enjoyment to a staff member's relationship with a person with dementia.

Greeting the Person and Improving Recognition

Depending on the severity of the dementia, the person may or may not recognize even a familiar staff member, family member, or friend. Without recognition, the opening moments of any interaction can be difficult. The person may become alarmed ("Who is this woman approaching me?"), embarrassed ("I should know this woman, but . . . "), or fearful ("I don't want him helping me dress!"). When the person's Life Story has been mastered by a Best Friends care partner, you can easily learn better ways to introduce yourself and establish an immediate connection.

Consider the following example. A day center bus driver who picks up a client at her home knows that the woman can sometimes be nervous and reluctant to leave. He starts the interaction by smiling, extending a warm handshake or touch, and introducing himself: "Hi, Mary! I'm John, your bus driver from the senior center." If John knows Mary's Life Story, he can add something such as, "I see you are wearing that pretty pink dress. I remember that pink has always been your favorite color." Then he might add, "How is your grandson, Ed? Is he still on the high school football team?" Happily, she now gets on the bus.

Introducing the Person to Others

In residential or day center settings, the person can be introduced with a biographical fact, such as, "I'd like you to meet my friend, Miles, who was born in London, England." In turn, you can say, "Miles, I'd like you meet Shirley. She's traveled to London many times." This old ritual helps make connections, builds self-esteem, and helps build real relationships between people.

During a group activity, staff can go around a circle or room and "reintroduce" everyone, each time adding some small piece of biographical information. For example, if the group is tossing a ball around a circle, the director of the activity can say something about each person who catches the ball, such as, "Okay, now the ball is for Joanne. Joanne has a granddaughter named Nawanta." These few words draw Joanne's attention to the activity and increase her interest in continuing to play the game. The fact that the day center director has something special to say about everyone as the activity progresses promotes individual self-esteem while building group cohesiveness.

Reminiscing

People with Alzheimer's disease still enjoy reminiscing. When looking at an old family photograph, the person may, with cuing, be able to recall some names and relationships. If not, the photograph can still be used to talk about fashions from that era ("Claire, look at the hats ladies used to wear!") or to discuss other interesting items in the photograph ("Claire, is that lady wearing a real fur coat?").

Memories and impressions of parents and grandparents often remain vivid.

> Rebecca Riley loved to tell the story of a gentle horse she was riding as a young girl, when something spooked the horse and it took off. She had quite a thrilling ride, but her grandparents were scared to death!

Early childhood stories, particularly ones that involve childhood mischievousness, are enjoyable to the person. Gently teasing a retired college professor about how he used to skip school can bring laughter. A day center participant can be reminded of the time he stuffed his uncle's wool hat up the chimney to hide it, only to be found out when a fire was lit and the room filled with smoke!

> Margaret Brubaker enjoyed being reminded (and teased) about the times she played the game of craps. She even taught her son Jim how to play. Because she always greeted visitors in such a proper manner and appeared to be very traditional, it was fun to reminisce with her about this unexpected talent.

Improving Communication Through Clues and Cues

The Life Story may provide clues to aid in understanding what the person is saying when wrong words or incomplete sentences are spoken. For example, if someone with dementia says, "I need to get home, the children, it's getting late," a staff member who is familiar with the person's Life Story might recall that she was a homemaker who made a big dinner for her family every night. The staff member might make a guess and say, "Oh, Carol, don't worry. I bet that your daughter Stephanie has already made a delicious dinner for everyone. Tonight *you* get to be spoiled."

The Life Story also helps us to provide clues, when needed, to allow the person to finish a sentence. If someone says, "I need to call my husband . . . " and is struggling to find his name, a staff member can supply the name by saying, "You mean your husband, Mike?" If someone keeps talking about his or her childhood but seems unable to supply many details, you can use the Life Story to inquire, "Mary, it must have been wonderful growing up in the pretty town of Walla Walla. Aren't you lucky to have grown up surrounded by those beautiful wheat fields and famous sweet onions?"

> Evelyn Talbott had an intense desire to converse. She lit up whenever someone prompted her about her work, her love of dogs, her interest in dancing, and her enjoyable nature walks. She used her hands to gesture toward her body, saying with her hands, "Give me more, keep going." People who knew elements of her Life Story found it easy to converse with her, but someone who did not know much about her would find the conversation ended quickly. Evelyn needed others to do most of the work, to "carry the ball" in conversations.

Designing Appropriate Activities

We can look to the person's Life Story for clues about past and present interests and skills. For example, an accountant diagnosed with Alzheimer's disease certainly will no longer be able to handle a complex transaction, but he or she might enjoy "helping" to add a row of figures. One could ask a retired librarian to help organize a collection of magazine clippings and photographs. A former homemaker may enjoy helping to prepare a batch of cookies or folding laundry. A retired shoe salesperson may enjoy looking at wholesale shoe catalogs and "placing" a new order. The possibilities are endless.

> Larkin Myers enjoyed teaching others how to "spin a top." He had retained his childhood skill of winding the string on the wooden top and then spinning it so it would whirl around for a seemingly impossible length of time.

The Life Story provides a rich source of ideas for show and tell. If the person had created crafts, collected stamps, painted, won bowling trophies, and so forth, the Life Story can note these experiences, which can then be used one-on-one to reminisce. Simply bringing in a collection of old neckties would probably fill an afternoon with discussion and laughter about the varying styles, colors, and widths that came into, out of, and back into fashion.

Pointing Out Past Accomplishments

We honor persons with dementia by remembering their accomplishments and the accomplishments of family members. Rebecca Riley, for example, loved it when you reminded her of her academic achievements or the time she successfully pulled off a dinner for 500 people.

The Life Story also gives us information to be able to point out the accomplishments of family members. For example, almost all parents like hearing good things about their children. We can point out when someone's grandson is the star football player or congratulate the person if his or her daughter has just received a big promotion.

Helping to Prevent Behavior that Is Challenging

Many challenges are caused by identifiable triggers, such as being exposed to grandchildren who are too loud, being asked inappropriate questions, or being rushed. However, sometimes behaviors may stem from more deep-rooted concerns that might be apparent only from the person's Life Story. For example, if a person lost family members in a boating accident, problems may occur if a volunteer in a day center shows photographs of his or her new boat. The person may not be able to explain his or her feelings and instead might leave an activity they usually enjoy or become despondent.

> Geri Greenway found popular music distasteful. She enjoyed fine classical music and opera but could not abide the popular, nostalgic songs often sung in the day program. Staff quickly learned to distract Geri and let her do other things during the music hour.

In Geri's case we learned to simply take her out of the room when the popular music began. Knowing her Life Story also allowed us to redirect her with something she loved: listening to her favorite opera or classical music. Sometimes one or two key "favorite things" from a Life Story can turn around a difficult situation.

Incorporating Past Daily Rituals

Because a ritual is a long-standing routine or habit, past daily rituals often still have meaning and can be used in dementia care. If a person enjoyed a daily newspaper, let him or her start the day that way. Even when the person may not be able to fully read a paper or retain the content, there is enormous symbolic value in simply holding it and turning the pages. Reading a newspaper suggests to others that one is educated, informed, and interested in the world.

If the person enjoyed a morning cup of coffee (or other beverage), make the most of this past ritual. Offering the person a cup of coffee prepared just the way he or she likes is a social interaction as well as a gift, and the coffee's warmth and aroma may stimulate positive memories.

Happy hours or afternoon teas can celebrate past rituals. Rituals can also include evening activities. For example, many assisted living programs show old episodes of *The Tonight Show* with Johnny Carson to wind down the evening.

Broadening the Caregiving Network and Resources

A Life Story can remind families, agencies, adult day center directors, and residential care community operators of the richness of the person's past. In many cases the person volunteered in church groups or civic and social clubs or belonged to a special military unit, the police or fire department, or a trade union.

Incorporating the Life Story into Your Care Setting

Rebecca Riley's Life Story in Chapter 1 celebrates her rich life and offers an example of how preparing a Life Story can be essential to dementia care. Many of the people you support have some similar Life Story elements to Rebecca Riley. How can you be a Best Friend to a person with dementia who, like Rebecca:

- was a nurse
- had a deep faith
- liked to be busy and productive
- grew up on her grandparents' farm
- was nominated for Mother of the Year
- loved gourmet cooking

With appropriate consent, the Life Story can be a great source of organizations or volunteers who can support your program. Can the local fire department bring its mascot dalmatian to the nursing home to visit a retired firefighter with dementia? Can a church organist play for a member who can no longer attend services, or can a local service club raise funds for a new adult day center that would benefit several of its members?

> Because the day center staff knew that Nancy Zechman was an avid tennis player, they looked to her social contacts and friends for potential volunteer help. Her tennis partners at the Lexington Tennis Club were contacted, and Nancy's close friend Jody Bollum agreed to be with Nancy at the day center once a week. When they were together, Jody helped Nancy feel safe and secure, in part because they had many stories and experiences in common. Other ladies from the club also lent their support, coming to the day program and regularly walking with Nancy.

Best Practices for Enhancing Preparation of the Life Story in Your Dementia Program

Despite our goals, we know that Life Stories sometimes just don't get written up or completed. We hope this chapter has inspired you to refocus on this key element of care. The important thing is to start somewhere. If you are a CNA or activity professional in a program that isn't preparing Life Stories well, create your own set of cards with facts about each person. Sometimes even knowing one or two key facts can help build a relationship.

Here are some further suggestions for revamping your preparation of the Life Story.

Make Sure Forms and Information Are Accessible

Does everyone know where the Life Story form is kept? Is the information gathered up front and shared with all before services begin? Make sure that this vital information doesn't get stuck in marketing or on a manager's desk. If you are a manager, consider having a Life Story scavenger hunt where staff have to find information in various charts or binders.

Freshen Up the Design of Your Life Story Form

Does your program have a nicely printed and designed Life Story form, or is it a simple Word document? Update your form and ask a designer or in-house talent to polish it. Giving your Life Story form or forms a new, fresh look can help everyone grasp that this is a priority. Figure 3.2 shows page 1 of very nicely designed and inviting Life Story forms courtesy of The Grove program of American Baptist Homes of the West (ABHOW).

Keep It Fresh

We recommend that a person's Life Story be updated regularly. Life carries on, and many of the people in your care setting will have new and updated information to include in the Life Story. Set aside time to see whether there have been any major family developments, such as weddings, reunions, or new grandchildren. Has the person gone on a trip? Has the family given the person a new pet? Have any of the person's preferences changed?

Consider taking the first week of every quarter to update all the Life Story forms in your program. Another approach is to update a person's Life Story form on his or her birthday. This works well because there may be family visitors or friends coming to the birthday; ask them for information and help. Use the occasion to learn some new things ("I didn't know he loved German chocolate cake so much!").

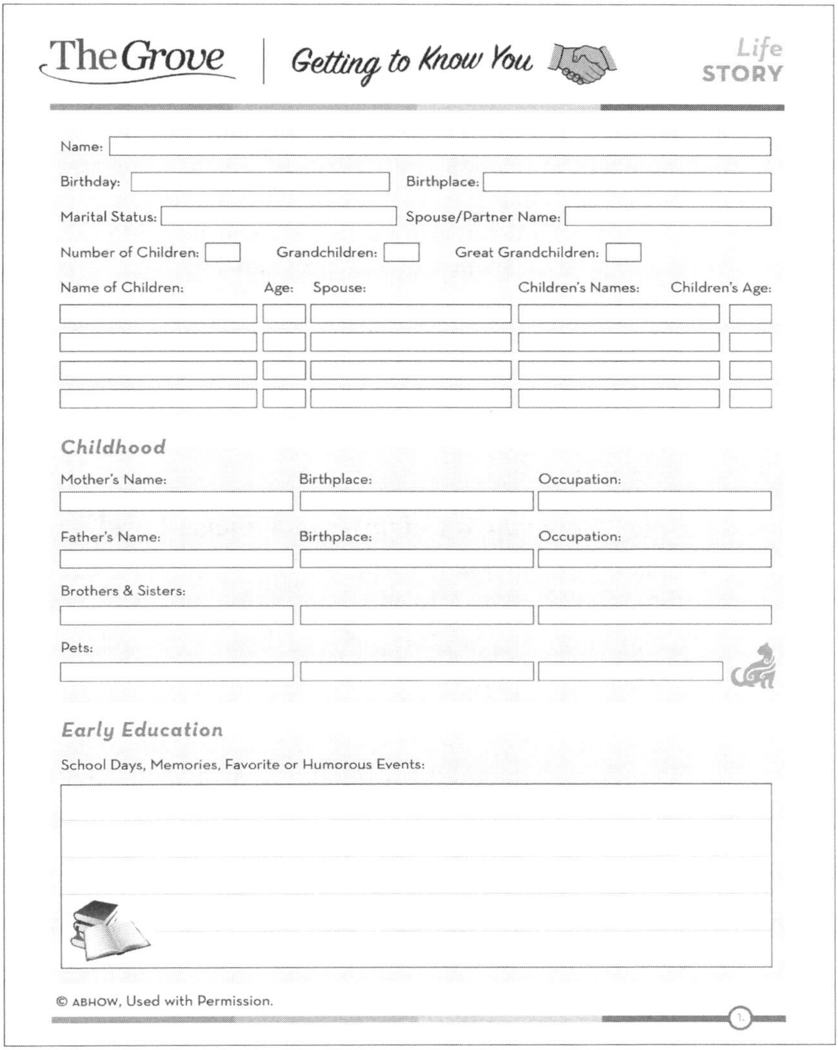

The Grove | Getting to Know You — Life STORY

Name:

Birthday: Birthplace:

Marital Status: Spouse/Partner Name:

Number of Children: Grandchildren: Great Grandchildren:

Name of Children:	Age:	Spouse:	Children's Names:	Children's Age:

Childhood

Mother's Name: Birthplace: Occupation:

Father's Name: Birthplace: Occupation:

Brothers & Sisters:

Pets:

Early Education

School Days, Memories, Favorite or Humorous Events:

© ABHOW, Used with Permission.

1.

Figure 3.2. ABHOW sample Life Story form (courtesy of The Grove program of American Baptist Homes of the West; used with permission).

Create a Top Ten Card or Form

Programs benefit from a comprehensive Life Story form, but sometimes you just need the essentials. Create a simple Best Friends Top Ten card, such as the one shown in Figure 3.3 for Virginia Bell, and distribute it to new staff members to quickly bring them up to speed or as a way to reinforce for existing staff the work of preparing and updating the Life Story. Creating the card can also be a good team-building exercise; create a work group to do them for your program or assign each staff member a person to write up.

Another good idea is to include the Top Ten card with someone in your care who is being hospitalized or going for a short-term nursing or rehab stay. This will give staff at the new setting important insights and also demonstrates to potential referral sources your commitment to high-quality dementia care.

Create a Display Honoring a Celebrity or Famous Local

Prestige Care reminds staff about the importance of the Life Story by maintaining a prominent display of 100 Things About John Wayne, Elvis Presley, Marilyn Monroe, or a local celebrity, such as a famous local college sports coach or historic figure. Discovering that the famous cowboy actor's real name was Marian, his nickname was the Duke, and he once dressed up as an Easter bunny for the television comedy *Laugh In* helps staff and families see how interesting it is to know a lot about someone.

Have a Resident or Person of the Week or Month

Select a resident of the week or month and ask care team members to learn all they can about the person. Create a bulletin board in the person's honor and enjoy all of the new material you have learned.

Create Trivia Games or Jeopardy

Use key facts about the people in your program in a game of Jeopardy or trivia contest with questions like "Who speaks five languages?" and "Who is famous for her homemade pies?" This reinforces information and adds some fun to our work in enriching the Life Story.

Discover the Life Stories of Your Staff

Have fun creating some Top Ten cards or learning Life Story highlights about the staff. We all love learning more about each other, and there are

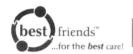

The Top Ten Things a Best Friend
Should Know About Me

Name: Virginia Bell   **Date:** 7-8-2014

1. Born on a farm in Kentucky.

2. Married to her husband Wayne, a retired minister and Seminary President.

3. Family oriented. Loves to talk about her extended family.

4. Always valued school and learning – got her Master's Degree at age 60.

5. Known for her home-made "cornpudding" recipe.

6. Proud of her career as a writer and Alzheimer's specialist.

7. Likes to be productive with meaningful engagement.

8. Has been to 40 countries for work and for play!

9. Enjoys a good cup of coffee (decaf, black) and one glass of wine before dinner

10. Won many first place awards for running in the Bluegrass 10 K race.

Figure 3.3.   Sample Top Ten card.

often some fun surprises (the receptionist drives a Harley motorcycle, or the chef is an old movie buff). Working with each other in gathering Life Story highlights creates a more cohesive team and a caring community. Staff will also connect the dots; they enjoy learning new things about each other, and this enjoyment carries over to learning new things about the person with dementia.

Conclusion

Good dementia care is individualized care, which is why the Life Story is a cornerstone of the Best Friends model of care. By using the Life Story, all staff members can help create special, caring, one-on-one relationships with persons with dementia, whether at home, in a day center, or even in a large nursing home.

If you work in a setting that is not fully on board with preparing and using the Life Story, remember that this is something you can do on your own. In just 5 minutes, you can learn a person's favorite color, foods, and music, whether he or she likes dogs or cats (or hates them!), and where he or she was born. Once you make these discoveries, use them throughout your day to engage the person. Share your findings with other staff members, and you will be taking a great step toward creating a caring community for all. As one staff member told us, "The more I give, the more I get." The person with dementia will value your interest and caring connection.

Creating a Life Story has another important value: it's a way of recording one's life achievements, both for the person with dementia and for his or her family. When families come together to create the document, the Life Story can be a healing tool. It can be a gift to give families after a loved one's death. It can be a document to be treasured for generations to come.

We hope that the information in this chapter will inspire you to review and refresh your approach to the personal and social histories of the people in your program. Let's bring the Life Story to life in your care setting!

CHAPTER 4

The Best Friends Approach to Communication

When you are a Best Friends care partner supporting persons with Alzheimer's disease or other dementia, communication can be perplexing and challenging. How do you keep someone engaged in conversation if she or he is losing the ability to communicate (sometimes caused by a condition known as *aphasia*), or can't remember what was just said? How do you encourage a person to take her medication, change into clean clothes, or drink some water to stay healthy? Is there a way to turn a *no* into a *yes*, particularly if you are trying to invite a person out of his room to come to an activity you know he will enjoy? The Best Friend staff understands that communication challenges are an everyday experience. As care partners, we believe that people still retain a desire to communicate long after their vocabulary and language skills diminish. They need us to keep trying with our words and actions.

We can't reverse the damage to the brain that is causing language skills to fail, but we can embrace the Best Friends™ approach to communication and learn strategies to stay connected to the person. In this chapter, you will see the Best Friends model applied to a number of brief, scripted scenes. Because the words we use have an impact on care, we conclude with some suggestions for changing the language we use to describe dementia.

How Best Friends Communicate

In any good friendship there is lots of communication. We talk to each other face to face and over the phone. We text or post on Facebook. We are tuned into our friends through body language. We may greet a friend with a hug and a friendly "hello." We roll our eyes when someone says something stupid or point to our watch when we want to leave early. When we are with a good friend, even silence can communicate a message; good friends can just look at each other and understand what is going on. Simply put, the Best Friends philosophy is that we as care partners need to make the effort to keep the person engaged in life. Even with communication losses, the person still retains a desire to communicate. We need to do all we can to fulfill this desire.

In good friendships, we compensate for areas of weakness in each other. Because the disease process has an impact on language, we cannot expect the person with dementia to do an equal share. That means that as a Best Friends care partner, you will need to do most of the work. And you can, by mastering the basics of communication and using tips that help communication go more smoothly, even in tense situations.

Master the Basics of Communication

First, cover the basics:

- Minimize distractions.
- Make eye contact, use gestures, and speak up.
- Listen actively.
- Pay attention to your nonverbal communication.
- Address the person as an adult.

Minimize Distractions

Is the home, day center, or residential home well lit, clean, uncluttered, and pleasant, or is it full of potential distractions? A messy, cluttered space can distract a person with dementia, reducing the ability to focus. Communication can also be challenged by constant bells and beeps from pagers, or pages from a public address system: "Sally, pick up line 3. Line 3 for Sally!" Work with your team to identify and eliminate "noise pollution." As Rebecca Riley once told us, "It is difficult to follow conversation with so much noise."

Make Eye Contact, Use Gestures, and Speak Up

Many older people have limited vision and poor hearing. Make sure that you are making eye contact (at least in most cultures), slow down, and (very important) speak up. Hand gestures (such as motioning a person to sit in a chair) can also support good communication.

Actively Listen

Work to be there for the person by actively listening. This means sitting near the person at the same level they are, taking a deep breath, slowing down, and giving the situation some time. Sometimes just waiting a minute longer for the person to answer creates a positive result. Waiting a moment is particularly critical for people who have been diagnosed with primary progressive aphasia (PPA), a form of cognitive impairment that involves a progressive loss of language function. As the parts of the brain responsible for speech and language degenerate, so does language function—even though other cognitive skills may be intact. Listening actively and waiting patiently for a response can help relieve the deep loss and frustration that persons with PPA feel.

Pay Attention to Your Nonverbal Communication

What are you communicating through your posture and facial expression? The person is looking for a friendly face, and your confidence and positive emotion will help the person relax and enjoy your time together. Conversely, a staff member who doesn't smile or comes to work in a bad mood is destined to face some struggles that day; people with dementia are sensitive to our moods.

Address the Person as an Adult

The person will sense if you are talking down to him or her or using childlike language. Avoid words that can be disrespectful, such as "sweetie" or "honey," and dumbed-down or baby talk. Don't exaggerate your speech, as in "My . . . name . . . is . . . Mary." It's better to speak in a normal pattern—"My name is Mary"—but slowly, and repeat the introduction if needed.

Interacting as a Best Friend

Use these tips to get a conversation off to a great start and affirm the person's connection with you:

• Always introduce yourself.
• Make a good first impression.

- Use the person's preferred name.
- Use positive language.
- Give lots of compliments.
- Ask for an opinion.
- Use the Life Story to improve conversation.
- Use repetition.
- Use good timing.
- Rely on humor.
- Don't take the person too literally.
- Give the person time to process and respond.
- Screen out troubling messages or news.

Always Introduce Yourself

It can also be helpful to introduce yourself, even if you regularly work with the person. For example, if you are working in-home, start the day by saying, "Good morning, Joan, it's your friend, David. It's great to spend some time with you."

Make a Good First Impression

First impressions are everything. Greet the person with a smile, enthusiasm, open arms, or a friendly handshake. Those opening moments can make the difference at the beginning of your shift or in the morning when encouraging the person to get up and have an enjoyable day. Helmut Graetz, a dedicated volunteer at the Best Friends™ Day Center, will sometimes "ham it up" with someone who is challenging. "I greet the person like I would a friend I have not seen in years with enthusiasm and joy. It usually turns things around, but occasionally I get a caustic look and know I've gone too far."

Use the Person's Preferred Name

Some programs still insist on using formal salutations like, "This is Mr. Jones" or "Miss Shirley." As a courtesy, always start with a more formal approach, but if the person says, "Call me Bob," you've been given permission to relate to him with his preferred name.

Does he want to be called Dr. Marks, Matt, or Pops? First names are meaningful in dementia care because the first name is probably our longest-held memory; our mothers and fathers used it when we were infants.

Use Positive Language

Whenever possible, speak to the person using positive language. It's better to say, "Let's go this way" than "Don't go that way." However tempting, never say, "I told you not to do that," or "No!" Persons with dementia are often proud, and no one likes being told what to do. Positive language also creates an emotional feeling that all is well, something that persons will respond to. Positive language also contributes to a culture of respect and caring.

Give Lots of Compliments

Compliments don't take much time (a minute or less) and don't cost any money. Telling a person with dementia that she looks lovely in her purple sweater or that she's the best teacher you've met lifts her up, creates smiles and feelings of satisfaction, and builds self-esteem. And if you're lucky, you'll get a compliment in return!

Ask for an Opinion

Asking someone for an opinion shows that you value the person and, as the Dementia Bill of Rights notes, understand that he or she has a point of view. A Best Friends staff member will often ask a person with dementia for some simple opinions: "Do you like my new hair color?" "Do you like my beard, or should I shave it off?" Be careful—the unvarnished truth is what you may get ("I don't like that beard at all!"). You can also ask for a person's opinion or lead a group discussion on some broader life issues. For example, "My boyfriend proposed, but we've only been dating 3 months—is that too soon?" This kind of question can often lead to meaningful discussion and even some friendly debate (e.g., whether it's best to wait a year to get married or to believe in "love at first sight" and go for it).

Use the Life Story to Improve Conversation

Using the Life Story helps improve communication in many ways. Knowing facts about the person helps you "fill in the blank" or provide other verbal cues. You can also bring up a favorite subject to show the person that you know him or her well. Sometimes knowing just one thing can help you start some positive communication: "How did it feel to be considered for Mother of the Year?" (one of Rebecca Riley's life achievements). Knowing the Life Story also helps us understand what the person is communicating. For example, when he or she mentions Miami Beach, it can be our cue to talk about favorite Cuban dishes.

"Shoe and Tell"

Do you have a team member who loves clothes or has dozens of purses and lots of shoes? Ask her to start a weekly tradition of bringing in a few fun outfits, two pairs of shoes, and several purses. The care partner can start the activity by say something like, "I have a date tonight. Can you help me put my outfit together?" When we've tried this activity in residential care, it has been a huge hit because it evokes old rituals (shopping with a girlfriend or helping your daughter get ready for an event) and makes people feel valued by asking for an opinion. "Shoe and Tell!" works well one-on-one or in a group setting.

Use Repetition

Best Friends staff understand that short-term memory loss contributes to miscommunication and that some gentle repetition helps. Asking a question twice, with additional descriptive cues for greater emphasis, can help the person better understand what care partners are saying: "Mrs. Smith, hand me that broom [pointing], please. Mrs. Smith, hand me that yellow broom over there [pointing]."

Use Good Timing

Get on the person's wavelength to know when to lend verbal assistance. For example, if waiting 15 seconds will allow him or her to complete a sentence, be patient (even when 15 seconds seems an eternity) and let the person enjoy success. If he or she is struggling, by listening carefully and drawing on your knowledge of the Life Story, you might be able to supply a missing word or phrase.

Rely on Humor

Sharing a joke or pun and a corresponding laugh is communication at its finest. It involves bonding and an emotional release. Also, laughter is infectious; we tend to laugh at a joke whether we get it or not. Best Friends™ Day Center participant Jerry Ruttenberg was part of an activity during which the group was talking about going to the beach. As part of a discussion about sand dollars, Virginia Bell asked, "I wonder how sand dollars reproduce?" Jerry quickly answered, "Maybe they have baby dimes."

Don't Take the Person Too Literally

Dementia affects word retrieval and vocabulary. The person may think he or she is being clear but may be using the wrong word, saying, for example, "Hand me that glass" while really meaning "coffee cup." Recognize that this is a challenge and take in the whole picture. Even if the person is using the wrong word, you may be able to easily figure out the message or request.

Give the Person Time to Process and Respond

In the busy work environment, we sometimes do our work quickly. In dementia care, that rarely helps; we need to slow down and be present for the person. If you are asking a person to do something or inviting him or her to an activity, be sure to allow time for processing and response. If you are patient, the person may answer your question or respond without you having to use a cue. And even if your intentions are good (preserving dignity), it can cause added frustration if you continually answer for the person.

Screen Out Troubling Messages or News

Because the person has difficulty sorting out information, it's important to screen out sad, violent, ominous, or controversial messages, when possible. Even distressing stories with a happy ending can cause a person to worry. For example, if a staff member tells the person that her car was stolen but found a few hours later, the person may get stuck in the middle of the story and continue to be concerned about the initial theft.

Communicating When Things Get Tough

These tips will help when you encounter difficulties:

- Realize that behaviors communicate a message.
- Try three times to turn a *no* into a *yes*.
- Do not argue or confront.
- Respond to emotional needs.
- Take the blame.
- Be affirming.

Realize that Behaviors Communicate a Message

Early in the disease, the person can communicate feelings and problems in words. Later on, his or her behavior articulates what words cannot. Behaviors such as yelling or striking out can signify that the person is in pain. Agitation can suggest boredom. Tears can suggest loneliness and the need for more activity and interaction with other people.

Try Three Times to Turn a *No* into a *Yes*

Persons with dementia inevitably say no to many things because they may not understand what you are asking, or they feel safer doing nothing.

> An innovative concept in the Home Instead Senior Care® network's dementia curriculum teaches its staff (called CAREGivers℠) to try "three times to turn a no into a yes." For example, a CAREGiver might invite a person to come out to the garden. If the person declines, the second request might involve describing the beautiful roses to spark interest. If the person again declines, the CAREGiver might now ask for help with watering or pruning the roses. Perhaps now the person will say yes.

Do Not Argue or Confront

It's virtually impossible to win an argument with a person with dementia. Trying to present an argument or to convince the person of a particular point of view will lead to frustration and failure. Also, confrontation only causes a person to be more defensive. So if the person says that you're late in serving him lunch (and you aren't), don't argue and correct him; instead say "I'm sorry." This apology (and a snack) de-escalates the situation.

Respond to Emotional Needs

The Dementia Bill of Rights includes the right "to be treated as an adult, listened to, and afforded respect for one's feelings and point of view." As care partners, we must work to understand the emotion behind unintelligible words. If the person seems upset, say, "I'm sorry about that," or when he or she seems happy, "That must have been great!" If the person can articulate concerns or feelings about his or her illness, validate and empathize with them ("It must be hard to have to leave your home after 40 years"). Comforting words or welcomed hugs can also make an emotional connection and provide reassurance.

The time may come when a person becomes completely nonverbal. Steve Troyer, a participant in the Best Friends™ Day Center, cannot speak, but he still has a need to express emotions and give opinions. With the help of staff and volunteers, he succeeds.

> Assistant Director Tracy Byrne drew from Steve's Life Story recently during a group discussion about names of sports teams throughout the country. Steve graduated from Purdue with a degree in mathematics, and school's sports teams are all named "the Boilermakers." Tracy addressed this question to him: "Steve, thumbs up or thumbs down—are you a Boilermaker?" With delight Steve gave a thumbs-up sign. This invitation to express himself makes Steve feel a part of the conversation.

Volunteer Lynda Woodard has used art to help Steve express his emotions. One day, after Lynda and Steve had played several games of Tic-Tac-Toe with pencil and paper, Steve took a new piece of paper and drew a face with a smile on it. He liked the game! But when a nurse told him he couldn't have a snack because his stomach had been upset, he took another sheet and drew a new face. In this picture, the mouth was a straight line and a tear fell from each eye. When Tracy Byrne saw it, she told him she had changed her mind and that he could have a snack. If the snack upset his stomach, they would just deal with it. He turned his thumb up and drew another face with a smile and no tears.

"How the person is perceiving his or her environment and the attitudes and actions of others will affect his or her ability to communicate and cope within that particular group," says Lynda. "I hope that we as Best Friends never assume that a person can't do something just because we haven't seen or heard him doing it before. The person may never again respond to that particular activity in the same way. But when a person does respond, for just that one moment we have connected. We never know when, where, or how that will happen, but seeking and finding those moments is the joy and mystery of sharing our hearts and time with our friend at Best Friends."

Take the Blame

Sometimes when things just aren't going well, it's a good idea to take the blame and apologize. "I'm sorry Joe, it's me not you, but I'm just not understanding. Let's try again." Saying you are sorry can also be a good response when the person is upset and you don't want to argue or correct the person. Follow your apology with a positive remark: "I'm glad we are still friends" or "I know you will forgive me since we are friends." This can smooth over rough waters and restore happiness and calm to the situation.

Be Affirming

If the person's words cannot be understood, make an affirming statement such as, "Doug, I always enjoy being with you" or "Miss Stevens, you usually have all the right ideas." Many persons can detect a lack of sincerity. Sometimes it's even okay to simply apologize and say, "I'm sorry I can't quite understand. Let's keep trying."

Communicating Skillfully

The following scenarios apply the Best Friends approach to some familiar communication challenges. Watch as Best Friends staff listen

The Best Friends Approach to Communication

- Minimize distractions.
- Make eye contact, use gestures, and speak up.
- Listen actively.
- Pay attention to nonverbal communication.
- Address the person as an adult.
- Always introduce yourself.
- Make a good first impression.
- Use the person's preferred name.
- Use positive language.
- Give lots of compliments.
- Ask for an opinion.
- Use the Life Story to improve conversation.
- Use repetition.
- Use good timing.
- Use humor.
- Don't take the person too literally.
- Screen out troubling messages or news.
- Realize that behaviors communicate a message.
- Try three times to turn a *no* into a *yes*.
- Do not argue or confront.
- Respond to emotional needs.
- Take the blame.
- Be affirming.

carefully, remain patient and empathetic, focus on the present, and use humor to bring a light touch to tough moments.

An In-Home Care Partner Asks Lance to Sit with Her

[Makes eye contact] *"Lance, come over here."*

[Gestures with hands and speaks in pleasant tone] *"Sit with me here on the sofa."* [Pats hand on sofa, smiling broadly]

"Come on, come into the living room, right here, this blue sofa is so comfortable. Good." [Gives a hug]

"I'm glad you're here beside me."

Note that the staff member speaks in short, direct sentences. She calls him by name, repeats key phrases, and uses gestures and body language effectively. Also, she adds emphasis when she mentions the sofa and then the "blue sofa." Then she gives him an affectionate hug, in a sense rewarding him for coming into the room.

Encouraging Involvement in a Simple Activity: Arranging Flowers

[Hands the day center participant, Jane, a vase of flowers] *"Jane, would you hold this pretty vase of flowers for me?"* [Gives her time to hold the small vase and admire the flowers]

"Would you put this orange vase [Gestures] *on that white table* [Points, gives Jane time to locate the table] *over there next to the piano?"*

"Help me organize this arrangement. [Asks for help] *Do you like the pink roses best or the yellow roses?"* [Asks for an opinion]

This next flower is beautiful. I get mixed up: Is it a tulip?" [Encourages Jane to process some simple information and respond]

Thank you for all your help; we've made this flower arrangement look its very best!"

The staff member used descriptive nouns instead of pronouns. She did not vaguely say, "Please put this over there." Instead, she talked about an orange vase and a white table next to the piano. She also showed patience by handing Jane the vase, letting her admire it, and taking time to let Jane see the table and the piano. In just a few sentences she captured many of the principles of communication discussed in this chapter. She asked for help (the person feels valued), she asked for an opinion about the flowers (helps the person feel in control), she encouraged Jane to respond about the type of flower (names of flowers like a tulip probably live in long-term memory), and she offered appreciation and thanks (something we all like).

Using Life Story Work to Have a Meaningful Talk About Art

[Gently takes the resident's hand and smiles] *"Good morning, Andrea. It's your friend, Mary. How are you this morning? I have a surprise for you!"* [Waits for response]

"I remembered that Pablo Picasso is your favorite artist. I brought this book in just for you. You know, I wish more people had an interest in art like you."

[Turning the pages] *"Do you like this portrait, or do you think it's too serious? I think she was one of his girlfriends!"*

The care partner cleverly inserts pieces of Andrea's biography (her interest in Picasso) into everyday conversation, making Andrea feel at ease and comfortable with a familiar friend. The fact that the day center staff member has individualized the activity to Andrea's past interests shows good use of Life Story information. The compliment she offers to Andrea ("I wish more people had an interest") seemed authentic and was probably appreciated. The last two sentences (asking an opinion and keeping a sense of humor) could lead to some playful discussion.

An In-Home Worker Coping with an Accusation

Joyce: [Angrily] *You took my purse! Where's my money?*

Jeff, care partner: [Keeps some distance, speaks in a calm voice, looks directly into Joyce's eyes] *Joyce, it's me, Jeff, your helper. I'm sorry that your purse is missing.* [Smiles] *Let me help you. I bet if we look together for a few minutes, we'll find that purse.*

Joyce: *Jeff, someone took my purse.*

Jeff: *Joyce, tell me about that purse. Is it the red one or the white one?*

Joyce: *It's my purse.*

Jeff: *I think I remember that you had the red purse out this morning. Was it the red purse?*

Joyce: *Yes.*

Jeff: *Here it is, Joyce. You know, I put it in the drawer for safekeeping. I'm very sorry if I upset you. I won't do it again.*

Joyce: *Well, okay. Don't touch it again.*

Jeff handles this situation well by keeping his distance initially and letting Joyce vent. He introduces himself and lets her know that he has taken her concerns seriously ("I'm sorry your purse is missing"). He then says that he put the purse away for safety reasons (which may or may not be true). He takes the blame for his client, smoothing over a difficult situation and helping her "save face" (protect her dignity).

Figuring Out Jumbled Words ("Word Soup")

Greg: [Looking agitated] *Oh! Oh! That's out. Cold.*

Linda: [Studies Greg's face, sees concern] *Greg, is something wrong?*

Greg: *It's cold. Noise. Cold.*

Linda: *It's cold outside. Let's look out the door. Will you help me take a look?* [Takes Greg by the hand and gently leads him to the sliding glass door] *Brrr, it's cold out there! Show me what you see.*

Greg: *There was noise.*

Linda: *Oh, are you looking at that cat out there? How did Bella get out? Shall we let him in? I think he likes you, Greg. Let's call him in and go sit together by the fire.*

Linda demonstrated effective communication by being patient, treating Greg's concerns as real, and piecing together the clues to discover that the cat had indeed gotten out in cold weather. By studying Greg's body language (his face and pacing), she determined that there was a problem and responded appropriately ("Is something wrong?"). Perhaps in this case she may also recall that Greg uses the word "noise" when he refers to the cat's "meow." Sometimes the puzzle can be solved.

Old Sayings

Many persons with dementia enjoy recalling old sayings. Have some fun by trying to name all of the old sayings that include an animal. Then ask the group what the old saying means. For example, "Why is a church mouse poor?" Find more on the Internet or in the "Old Sayings" activity in the *Best Friends Book of Alzheimer's Activities, Volume 1.*

- Crazy like a fox
- It's raining cats and dogs
- As poor as a church mouse
- A cat has nine lives
- A bird in hand is worth two in the bush
- Gentle as a lamb
- Cat got your tongue
- Hold your horses
- You can lead a horse to water, but you can't make him drink

Providing Emotional Reassurance Even when You Can't Follow the Words

Marsha, care partner: [Passing by Mrs. Arthur in the hallway] *Hello, Mrs. Arthur, I'm Marsha. It's nice to see you again. How is that sweet grandson of yours, Mike?*

Mrs. Arthur: *It's just, just there. Do that for me!*

Marsha: *Show me what you mean, Mrs. Arthur.*

Mrs. Arthur: *Do that.*

Marsha: [Not understanding] *You know, Mrs. Arthur, I enjoy being with you.* [Smiling] *I bet you are very wise about life. I could probably learn a lot from you!*

Mrs. Arthur: [Smiles and moves on down the hallway]

Marsha made the best out of a challenging situation. She greeted Mrs. Arthur cheerfully and recalled a fact from her Life Story to make a connection. Yet Mrs. Arthur's verbal skills have declined to the point that it's difficult to understand what she is saying. In this case, an affirmative statement, "I bet you are very wise about life," and then the compliment "I could probably learn a lot from you!" demonstrate respect and affection. Even though the statements stretch the truth a bit, they are said with caregiving integrity.

When you cannot figure words out, we suggest reading the emotion on the person's face and listening to tone of voice. In the above situation, it's okay to say, "I'm sorry, Mrs. Arthur, I don't follow what you are saying. Let's sit together and make sure everything is okay." The person may still be frustrated, but at least she feels you are on her side and trying to help.

Apologizing to Calm a Person's Anger

Sam, care partner: *Good afternoon, Pauline. It's great to see you looking so well. I brought your medications.*

Pauline, resident: *I am so angry with you. I've been waiting for hours. You are late, late, late!*

Sam: [Who isn't late] *Oh, my gosh, Pauline, the traffic was so bad today. I'm sorry that I'm late. I'll do better next time.* [Turns on his best charm and gives her a wink] *Will you forgive me?*

Pauline: *Okay, but shape up!*

Sam: *I will!*

Sam wasn't late, so it would have been easy for him to "defend himself" and correct her. But does it really accomplish anything to prove that Pauline is wrong and he is right? Doing this almost reinforces her cognitive losses by embarrassing and confusing her. By simply apologizing and then (with a wink) asking for forgiveness, Sam has defused the situation.

Changing a Wet Brief

Mylissa, in-home care partner: *It's almost time for lunch, Glenn. Let me help you clean up and get ready for lunch.*

Glenn: *I don't need any help.*

Mylissa: *I think your brief is wet. I know it's hard for you to feel that sometimes. The new fancy ones you wear are super absorbent.*

Glenn: *I'm not wet.*

Mylissa: [Approaching Glenn with a smile and open arms] *You are probably right, but it's worth checking. We want to get all freshened up to go out later to your favorite ice cream shop.* [Gently begins to encourage him to sit in the chair in his bedroom to get the personal care accomplished]

Glenn: *Is that the ice cream shop on Main Street?*

Mylissa: *Yes.* [Starts the process] *Oh my goodness, Glenn. This fooled both of us. Yep, I think we should put on a fresh, dry pair so you'll be more comfortable.*

Glenn: *Okay.*

Sometimes a person with dementia like Glenn will automatically say no to something when he does not quite understand what is being asked, or in this case, may not realize that the brief is wet. The care partner showed empathy by not embarrassing her client or treating him like a child (and note that she used the more dignified word *brief* instead of *diaper* or *Depends™*). Rather than argue, she gently coaxed Glenn and changed his mood by mentioning some favorite foods and an outing. Her body language and confidence helped turn that *no* into a *yes*. We also like the fact that her language was simple and direct.

Conclusion

Wouldn't it be great if besides preventing, slowing the progress of, or finding a cure for Alzheimer's and other dementias, we could also discover a medicine that preserved language? We would still have to cope with short-term forgetfulness, but life would be richer (and care easier) if we could fully understand the person and he or she could fully understand us. Until then, the Best Friends approach to communication will give you tools to bring out the best in the person with dementia.

When you go to work tomorrow, choose one person in your care setting and draw on the techniques in this chapter to be a Best Friend—to be present, to connect, and to use positive and affirming language. Hopefully, you will make a genuine connection that feeds your spirit and helps you better cope with the sometimes tough demands of your day. As we noted earlier, sometimes one good moment can last the whole day. Using the Best Friends approach to communication, we hope you will have many, many great days.

Now, in the next chapter, let's learn more about the Knack of great care and the art of doing difficult things with ease.

CHAPTER 5

The Knack

Dementia care has been a major focus in long-term care settings for many years now, yet programs still struggle to get dementia care right. Staff tell us that:

- Personal care is a struggle.
- We know we should be using the Life Story, but it just isn't happening.
- The activity program is flat; not enough is going on.
- Family complaints continue.
- Issues around wandering or elopement are arising.
- Turnover is high; staff are burning out.
- Behaviors are hard to understand and manage.

We also meet care partners who seem to have a magic touch in their relationships with people with dementia:

- The beloved nursing assistant who can rise to any occasion and always seems to say or do the right thing
- The day center activities director who implements ideas for a consistently rich and innovative program
- A waiter in senior living who gently gives some menu cues and suggestions to a resident having trouble navigating a menu
- The staff member who gets the showers done without a struggle
- The program administrator who creates an impromptu fashion show with her fun and colorful wardrobe

The difference between struggle and ease—the secret these staff members have mastered—is the Knack of care. Knack is all about delivering dementia care at its best. The word *knack* is defined as a clever trick or strategy or the "art of doing difficult things with ease." When you embrace the Best Friends™ approach and routinely ask yourself, "How can I be a Best Friend to this person?," the Knack will begin to become second nature.

Some lucky staff members are simply born with Knack. Their personality and sensibility help them to be wonderful care partners. For the rest of us, Knack is a skill set we can acquire. Knack brings together all of the core elements of Best Friends care into play. It's the whole package, expressed in a single word. As we understand and apply the dos and don'ts of Best Friends care, we start to embody the Knack—and offer excellent dementia care.

Elements of Knack

- Be well informed
- Have empathy
- Respect the basic rights of the person
- Have integrity
- Use common sense
- Communicate skillfully
- Maintain optimism
- Set realistic expectations
- Use humor
- Use spontaneity
- Maintain patience
- Develop flexibility
- Stay focused
- Be nonjudgmental
- Value the moment
- Maintain self-confidence
- Use cuing tied to the Life Story
- Take care of oneself

Elements of Knack

As Best Friends care partners, we strive to embody the elements of Knack described here and listed in the sidebar "Elements of Knack." Embodying all of the elements would be downright impossible, but learning and embracing even a few key elements can transform our work and help us become outstanding dementia care professionals.

Be Well Informed

Best Friends care partners with Knack learn as much as they can about dementia. They attend conferences and workshops, subscribe to appropriate newsletters, and talk to families coping with dementia. They actively seek to learn from other team members, including clinical staff. They know that the more one knows about dementia, the less stressful the difficult job of being a care partner can be. As noted in the Dementia Bill of Rights, a person has the right to care partners who are well trained in dementia care.

Have Empathy

Best Friends care partners with Knack have taken time to imagine what it would be like to have dementia. This helps them understand the world of the person they care for and how that world can be difficult and frightening. When we have empathy for a person with dementia, we grow to be forgiving and understanding of the bad days. Empathy also helps us develop strategies to overcome challenges and improve quality of life. For example, if we understand that a person accusing us of having taken his wallet is being forgetful, we can avoid overreacting and instead help him find the wallet. We can even share a laugh when we find it under the pillow.

Respect the Basic Rights of the Person

Best Friends care partners with Knack regard persons with dementia as human beings with infinite value who deserve loving, high-quality care. They embrace the spirit of the Dementia Bill of Rights by giving the person as much say in her care as possible and trying to keep her productive in purposeful chores and activity for as long as possible.

Have Integrity

Best Friends care partners with Knack act in the best interests of persons with dementia in their care by being real and authentic. They embody integrity by being honest and open with co-workers and treating a person like Rebecca as they themselves would want to be treated.

Use Common Sense

Best Friends care partners with Knack exercise common sense. That means, for example, eliminating caffeine when a person has problems sleeping, having a person wear an identification bracelet, and making extra photographs of a person if he or she is likely to leave a care setting. Common sense also reminds us to look for urinary tract infections, pain, or illness if a person with dementia has a sudden change in behavior, or to convene a Three New Ideas meeting to brainstorm new approaches to the situation (described in Chapter 7).

Communicate Skillfully

Best Friends care partners with Knack do their best to keep communication going, despite the cognitive losses of dementia. It's important to learn ways to communicate skillfully, slowing down and speaking up, cuing the person with appropriate words from his or her Life Story, using positive body language, and knowing the right and wrong ways to ask and answer questions. Looking at the person's facial expressions, listening carefully to their words, and paying attention to their actions also make a difference.

Maintain Optimism

Best Friends care partners with Knack look beyond the cognitive losses of dementia and focus on the positive. They smile, use upbeat language, and have good energy. When staff greet a person with comments like "It's going to be a wonderful day" (as opposed to, "It looks like a storm is headed this way!"), it sets the day up for success. Optimism also suggests that the behaviors that are so tough today may diminish or go away with the passage of time.

Set Realistic Expectations

Best Friends care partners with Knack have given thought to what the person can still do but don't expect so much as to cause frustration.

For example, a staff member who sets realistic expectations might encourage a musician with dementia to play a simple piano piece (helping him or her feel a sense of accomplishment), but would not ask the person to play something too complex (that might lead to failure and frustration). Staff with Knack strike just the right balance.

Use Humor

Best Friends care partners with Knack are not afraid to tell funny stories and jokes or laugh when humorous things happen. They understand that even when the person does not get a funny story or joke, laughter and good feelings are contagious. The person will absorb these good feelings. Another key element of humor is that care partners should not be afraid to make fun of themselves. Self-deprecation preserves dignity and is a small price to pay to make the person feel better about his or her own circumstances. These care partners don't mind sharing about the time they forgot to turn on the oven for the Thanksgiving turkey or put a sweater on backwards at the church social.

Use Spontaneity

Best Friends care partners with Knack are not afraid to be spontaneous. A day planned for planting vegetables might also include an hour of unplanned bird-watching when colorful cardinals are spotted in the trees. Persons with dementia live in a world full of spontaneous events. If the person becomes interested in the color of a car or a particular object in the house, go with the flow!

Maintain Patience

Best Friends care partners with Knack realize that it takes the person longer to do things and longer to respond to words and events. Bathing, grooming, and dressing can take 45 minutes, but during those 45 minutes the person is focused and does not feel lost or lonely. Getting frustrated or rushing the person only makes matters worse.

Develop Flexibility

Best Friends care partners with Knack recognize that the best-planned schedule cannot be set in stone because the person may have his or her own ideas about how the day will transpire. The person doesn't have to eat, take a shower, or go to bed on our schedule. The schedule is just a starting point; be flexible and let the person decide what he wants to do and when he wants to do it. In the best programs, we adapt to the person's needs. Why not give the shower after dinner instead of before breakfast?

Stay Focused

Best Friends care partners with Knack learn the importance of focus. With all of the distractions around us, it can be hard at times to give the person the attention needed to provide good care. This is particularly challenging in long-term care and day center settings, where many things are happening at once. A nursing assistant, for example, should always focus on giving someone a bath, not on talking about how a friend did not show up for a date. The Knack of focus involves really listening to and seeing the person as well as getting the most out of every interaction.

Be Nonjudgmental

Best Friends care partners with Knack work on being nonjudgmental toward the person, families, and each other. Many of our families have struggled for years before using services; it's important not to judge them for their actions or decisions. Similarly, we can't take sides in family disputes. We rarely know the whole story, and we want to be welcoming to all family members. Within our own work settings, team members will sometimes be at their best and other times let us down. Let's be forgiving and supportive of our team whenever possible while also maintaining a professional environment.

Value the Moment

Best Friends care partners with Knack know the importance of living in and valuing the moment. A pleasant lunch, time spent arranging flowers, or a joyful game may soon be forgotten, but it can be pleasurable for everyone in the moment. Be present for the person; give her your full attention. Say some simple words like, "I understand" or "I'm here for you." If care partners can learn to string together these positive moments, good dementia care can be achieved.

Maintain Self-Confidence

Best Friends care partners with Knack maintain self-confidence in their interactions with persons with dementia. (And we hope that the Best

Friends Approach will help give you this confidence!) To be confident, we need to feel that we know what we are doing, have a plan of action, and have some successes to make us feel that we are doing the right thing. This inner strength often can be sensed by the person, who may then let go of his or her own concerns or fears.

Use Cuing Tied to the Life Story

Best Friends care partners with Knack are able to incorporate the Life Story into all aspects of care, cuing the person to remember certain names, places, and things; telling familiar stories; and reminding her of past achievements. Sometimes just knowing a few favorite subjects can make everything better. Perhaps the person enjoys talking about her childhood in Santa Barbara or his college days at Tulane. Using the Life Story can also help us better understand behavior (the person has never liked crowds) and teach us subjects to avoid (a war experience or loss of a child).

Take Care of Oneself

It's hard to be fully present and helpful for others if you are not taking care of yourself. Just like the safety video shown on airplanes (you need to secure your own oxygen mask before helping someone else put on his or her mask), you have to devote time and effort to taking care of yourself if you are a care partner to others.

Best Friends care partners with Knack take time to exercise and eat well, pause to breathe deeply, and work to manage stress. We also encourage program leaders to maintain a commitment to a positive and successful workplace culture, with adequate resources to help staff succeed. It's hard to be there for our team and families if we aren't taking care of ourselves, too.

Knack in Dementia Care

The following scenarios show Knack at work in situations that commonly arise between staff and people with dementia. As you compare the "no-Knack" and "Knack" approaches, you'll see the Best Friends model in action. We know that most staff have great common sense and do the right thing, but we've exaggerated the "no-Knack" situations to add some humor and drive home our points (although not all of them are that exaggerated). May these examples inspire you to

The Knack, Canada Style

The Alzheimer's Society of Calgary has a strong focus on professional education. Its licensed Best Friends training curriculum uses the word *knack* as a clever acronym to teach the core Best Friends concepts:

- **K**nowledge (of the disease and the experience of the person with dementia)
- **N**urturing (by knowing the Life Story, making care relevant to each person)
- **A**pproach (practicing effective communication)
- **C**ommunity (facilitating activities with engagement)
- **K**inship (including friends and families in the care team)

Teaching and talking about Knack in this way brings the elements all together and helps staff visualize the idea of Knack and put it into practice in their daily work.

apply the lessons to your own setting. The result is dementia care at its best.

The Big Cat

A woman with Lewy body dementia approaches her in-home staff care partner in the family room looking upset and claims, "There's a big cat in my bedroom. He may hurt me!"

No-Knack Approach

"I bet it's one of those friendly circus animals. They can be really big, but I know how to tame them. Let me get some magic big cat food that I keep in the refrigerator. It will definitely tame him so we can all go to bed later tonight." [Moments later] *"I just went into the room and we talked and he went back to the circus."*

Example of Knack

"You stay here, Maggie, and I'll check out the room." [Moments later] *"Well, Maggie, I have some really good news. Everything is okay now! Maybe he jumped out of the open window. What a rascal! I think that cat might have been having fun at our expense. In any case, I've locked up so he can't get back in."*

Discussion

Sometimes people with Lewy body dementia will hallucinate and see people, animals, or other objects that are not present. In this scenario, it's not advisable to embellish the situation to a fantastic level (the circus animal, magic cat food), as was done in the no-Knack example. By taking Maggie's worries to such an extreme, the care partner was not respecting her fears and almost treated her like a child. Maggie may sense his lack of sincerity. Using the more low-key, matter-of-fact Knack approach ("I'll check out the room") provides a strong indicator that all is well, feels more adult, offers a sensible solution, and shows that the care partner listened.

We like the care partner's use of an old-fashioned word, "rascal," to describe what might have been this mischievous cat. This playful word used with a bit of humor communicates to the resident that all is well. Maybe the cat just wanted to make friends!

I'm Out of Here

A resident in memory care stands by the exit door saying, "I want to go home. I'm out of here!"

No-Knack Approach

[With impatience] *"This is your home! You live here now. Come with me. You are not allowed to stand at that door."*

Example of Knack

[Takes his hand and speaks calmly] *"Tell me about your home. Do you live in the city or country? Is it a nice house?"* This is also a great time to use the Life Story. For example, if you know the resident worked for the famous airplane manufacturer Boeing in Seattle, you can ask him, "Is it true that you helped design one of the biggest planes in the world? Tell me more about that."

Discussion

The person may think he's not at home, or he may not be speaking literally. Needing to go home may mean getting back to where things make sense again. The first response was argumentative (how many of us like to be told we are wrong?) and probably would have added to the resident's agitation.

The approach with the Knack showed sensitivity and listening skills. She asked about his home, which demonstrated that she was taking his concern seriously. By asking an open-ended question, she encouraged him to talk more about his feelings of home, if he wants to. Later, she used the Life Story to bring up a favorite subject and memory: working at Boeing. This gently redirected him away from his concern about home to a subject he likes to talk about.

Nobody Loves Me

Staff at the adult day center notice that one of their favorite participants seems teary-eyed and unhappy. Normally she enjoys all of the activities, including dancing and singing. "I'm very sad today. Nobody loves me anymore," is her reply when asked about her feelings.

No-Knack Approach

"I don't think it's good to feel sorry for yourself. You've got so much to be thankful for. You've got lots of family, including your granddaughter in Taiwan who is visiting you soon, your cousins in Ohio, and your sister in New York. You were happy yesterday; just try to enjoy yourself today."

Example of Knack

"I'm sorry you're feeling blue. I feel that way now and then, too." [Pauses for her to respond] *"But you know you are my friend and I love you a whole bunch."* [Pauses for a big hug and time together] *"Your granddaughter will be coming soon. That should be lots of fun."*

Discussion

The first response does not acknowledge the person's feelings. However well meaning, the staff member presented too much information all at once. Worse, she tried to explain away the problem and argue a different point of view. It's almost always impossible to win an argument with someone with dementia. The final statement, wherein the staff member simply ended the conversation by saying, in effect, "Shape up!," probably would not be helpful in any situation in which someone is feeling blue.

The approach with Knack affirmed the person's feelings of loneliness—not judging, just listening and accepting. The day center staff member admitted having similar feelings, which helps the person feel that she is not alone, that these feelings happen to all of us. The staff member responded in the present, letting the person know that she has one good, caring friend.

The staff member also masterfully used moments of silence to give the person time to respond. A big hug after a compliment also creates a special connection. Knowing the person's Life Story, the day center staff member is aware that the granddaughter is very special to this participant. She, therefore, reminds the woman that her granddaughter will be visiting soon, which gives her a good feeling.

It's Getting Late

Many adult day centers have participants who become worried late in the day. For example, they may be worried about who will pick them up, particularly if they see others going home on a busy day or being picked up by their family members.

No-Knack Approach

"It will be at least 2 more hours before your son comes, maybe more. You know he's very busy and sometimes runs late. Just relax!"

Example of Knack

"We are in touch with your son. He'll be here after we sing together. He'll be here soon."

Discussion

The first approach had several mistakes. First, giving too many details and trying to explain things logically add to the confusion and will not be remembered. Second, being too literal ("at least 2 hours") is also a recipe for disaster, particularly because many people with memory loss cannot keep track of the passage of time. Finally, mentioning that the son is often late suggests to the person that something is wrong, causing her to worry more.

The response with Knack is reassuring: "We are in touch with your son," and "he'll be here soon." Note that this stretches the truth somewhat, but still passes the integrity test. Adult day centers are usually able to reach family members when needed ("we are in touch"), and the word "soon" can be any length of time. In this case, the words are being used in the best interest of the person, to calm fears.

Distraction is also put into play to calm the person. The person's Life Story suggests an enjoyment of singing, so the mention of that part of the day evokes a smile and good feelings, which replace the anxiety.

I'm Late for an Appointment

Sometimes persons with dementia become worried or fixated on a certain event, even declining a meal or favorite activity because of that concern. One woman often worried about medical appointments, saying, "I'm late for an appointment." The frustrated staff often found her waiting by the door instead of participating in an enjoyable program.

No-Knack Approach

"Your appointment was canceled. Your doctor had to see a patient at the hospital. But don't worry, we're going to have fun today. The music starts at 3 o'clock."

Example of Knack

"Let me check on that appointment. I know that getting the job done and keeping your commitments is so important to you. [Takes a minute or two to pause and returns] *Oh, my gosh, that appointment isn't today. We will find out more about it. Meanwhile, I could sure use your help. Would you please help me get the room ready for the afternoon concert? We have your favorite country-western music today. You are my best assistant!"*

Discussion

This scenario is a good example of the subtleties of tying one's approach to the person's needs and special issues. The first response, wherein the staff member fibs about the appointment and immediately tries to gently cajole her into participating in the activity, was certainly friendly and well intentioned, but it did not respect her desire to keep her appointment.

In the approach with Knack, the staff member didn't just create a false story about the appointment. Instead she simply said that the appointment wasn't today—a response appropriate to the contemporary view of dementia care, which includes as much authenticity as possible.

The Knack approach also used a tried-and-true strategy: asking the person to help. Many persons with dementia enjoy being needed and productive.

The Solar System Can Wait Another Day

The program director worked with a college student volunteer to create an ambitious art project involving a mobile of the solar system. Balloons would be covered with papier-mâché strips and then painted to represent each planet.

On the big day, staff and volunteers gathered together. The director was ready with paper strips and glue. The balloons were colorful, and it was fun blowing them up to different sizes. Suddenly, one program participant batted a balloon in the air, another batted it back, and an extended balloon toss game was under way.

No-Knack Approach

"Let's stop this now! We must get this project finished. Next Tuesday is the day to paint the planets. If we don't get everything done today, we won't be ready. The planets need a week to dry."

Example of Knack

"What fun! Balloons are made for celebrations. I guess the solar system won't change between now and next week if we do the next part of the project later. You know what they say about the best-laid plans! Julia, hit Jupiter into the air!"

Discussion

Despite our program schedules, sometimes persons with dementia have their own ideas! They live and find joy in the moment. The best programs allow the residents to guide the flow of the day and weigh in on their likes and dislikes.

In this case, the day center director with no Knack was frustrated that she would fall behind schedule on her planetary project. Pushing the participants to move on could create tension and frustration. Would they have gotten any more joy from the completed project than from their spontaneous balloon toss?

The staff member with Knack was not afraid to laugh at herself ("the best-laid plans"). In this case, the approach with Knack was to take pleasure in the moment and to complete the papier-mâché project later. Activities with Knack do not focus too much on the end product; the process is just as important.

Let's Go to My Room and Fool Around

A person with dementia may mistake a staff member for his spouse. He suggests that they go to his room to "fool around."

No-Knack Approach

[Agitated] *"Shame on you, Joe. You are a married man. I'm going to tell your wife!"*

Example of Knack

[Calmly redirecting] *"Hey, Joe, it's Louise, your helper. Your beautiful wife, Joanna, should be here soon* [Shows him a picture of his wife that is in the room]*."*

Discussion

One quality to strive for in dementia care is being calm and collected when challenges arise. In this case, the person may be genuinely confused about identity. He may think that the staff member is his wife, and because of this mistake, his sexual advance does not seem so out of the ordinary. The first approach was done from emotion and shaming (and a probable lack of understanding about dementia care) and is certainly not successful.

The response with Knack is a sensitive one in so many ways. The staff member calmly reintroduced herself and cued him about his wife. She also showed him a framed picture of his wife and offered a compliment about the picture.

It's also important to note that sometimes the label of sexual inappropriateness is applied incorrectly. If a person begins undressing, it might be because he is too warm. A man might unzip his pants to go to the bathroom, not to expose himself.

We discuss more about sexuality in Chapter 7, "Best Friends and Behavior."

The More You Push, the More I'm Going to Push Back

A staff member is determined to get Mrs. Tucker to take her medications. She first offers Mrs. Tucker her pills, and she declines. "It's doctor's orders," the staff member says, picks up Mrs. Tucker's hand, and tries to get the pills in her palm. Mrs. Tucker reacts angrily and begins pushing the staff member away.

No-Knack Approach

[Tries to hold her down or hold her arms] *"Mrs. Tucker, don't get angry at me! I'm trying to help you! Stop that!"*

Example of Knack

[Staff member approaches Mrs. Tucker, knowing she is often reluctant to take her pills] *"I'm so happy to see you. You look so beautiful. I have your pills from the doctor. Do you want to take them now or after lunch?"*

Discussion

Behavior communicates a message. Most persons with dementia don't strike out randomly or have ongoing anger. When a person does strike out, it may be that we've accidentally triggered the response, perhaps by rushing the person. The more we push, the more a person pushes back.

The best generals know when to charge ahead and when to retreat. In the no-Knack scenario, the staff member lost her cool and used some very demeaning language ("Stop that!"). The care partner with Knack slowed down, gave a compliment, and offered Mrs. Tucker a simple choice. With any luck, she will feel more in control and readily take her medications (even if it's after lunch).

What Time Is It? What Time Is It?

Persons with dementia often repeat questions or requests, which can be extremely annoying to staff and other people in day center or residential settings. A typical situation might be when a person asks, "What time is it?" over and over again.

No-Knack Approach

"How many times do I have to tell you that it's 11:30 in the morning!"

Example of Knack

[Even if you just answered a few minutes earlier] *"Henry, it's 11:30 in the morning. Almost time for lunch. How can I help you? Are you worried about something? Here's a piece of fruit to tide you over."*

Discussion

It's only human to lose your patience, but in dementia care losing your cool typically escalates the situation. Repetition comes with dementia because of the damage to the brain's short-term memory functions. It can also represent unmet needs or anxiety.

The no-Knack approach focused on the answer to a question instead of underlying needs. Even if you had the patience to answer the question 30 times, it probably wouldn't help.

The example with Knack worked because the staff member looked beneath the words and tried to address the person's needs. The staff member also took the time to ask why he was anxious. Offering a favorite piece of fruit also set a good tone.

That's My Coat

Sometimes persons with dementia will pick up something belonging to someone else, most often because they think it's their property.

No-Knack Approach

"Mrs. Owens, that does not belong to you. Take that back where you found it!"

Example of Knack

"Why, Mrs. McArdle, you found my blue coat I misplaced. Thanks so much for returning it." [Then the staff member gently returns the coat to the owner's room]

Discussion

The no-Knack approach, most readers would agree, is wrong in many ways! The resident probably thinks it is her coat. Simply telling her it is not might create feelings of confusion, anger, or even distrust and suspicion. Even if the resident agrees to return it, she may not recall where it comes from.

The approach with Knack is simple and evokes old social graces to thank someone for a favor, in this case finding a "lost coat." If this approach does not work, we recommend that a staff member simply take the coat back while Mrs. McArdle is not looking or is involved in something else. Keep the environment simple and clutter free. If care partners can dispose of unneeded or unused possessions, it can make it easier to keep things in their proper place.

Ringing the Doorbell

In-home workers sometimes visit and support persons with dementia who still live on their own. The person may or may not remember that the family has hired some help, and some days he or she may resist having someone come in and help.

No-Knack Approach

Sylvia rings Mrs. Singh's doorbell. Mrs. Singh answers but looks from behind the screen door. "Hi, Mrs. Singh, it's Carmen, your staff person from the agency. I'm here to help you out and be sure you've taken your medications."

Mrs. Singh says, "No thank you. I don't need any help," and closes the door in Sylvia's face.

Example of Knack

As Mrs. Singh opens the door, the staff member smiles broadly and says, "Good morning. It's your friend Sylvia. I happened to be in the neighborhood and thought I'd drop by. I am friends with your son Paul. I'd love to come and work those crossword puzzles with you. May I come in?"

Discussion

Many persons with dementia remain quite proud. They don't want someone in their home even when they need help badly. They also worry about money, not believing that they can afford help (even if they can or the children are paying).

The no-Knack approach was too business-like and literal. "I'm here to help" may be true, but it sets up a dependency and unequal relationship; it's certainly not a care partnership.

The second approach with Knack seemed like a neighbor dropping by to help. The staff member used her knowledge of the Life Story to ask Mrs. Singh about a favorite activity of crossword puzzles. Once inside, Sylvia may be able to help Mrs. Singh take her medications and complete other chores.

Conclusion

One of our most memorable encounters was during a conference in Amsterdam, when we met a Dutch woman who described the essential qualities of good staff. "For my dementia program, I look for former barmaids and beauticians!" she said. We're still not sure whether she was pulling our leg, but we loved this idea! Bartenders and beauticians have qualities that we want in dementia care. They are good listeners, they are good storytellers, they cater to people's preferences, and they tend to be upbeat, positive people. Virginia Bell and David Troxel actually have met many wonderful staff members who were once bartenders or beauticians.

Kay Kallander, formerly senior vice president of strategic planning of ABHOW, often says, "When looking for staff, hire for the heart, train for the task." In other words, a staff member's personality, affection, patience, and heart—their Knack—is what counts the most.

And there's another benefit of the Knack. It's a strategy for success— not just a way to be nice and friendly. When the person trusts you, feels some control over his or her life, is active and engaged, and is in the relationship, you may experience fewer behaviors that are challenging and more cooperation. A Best Friends relationship is well under way.

CHAPTER 6

The Calendar Is Just the Beginning

Celebrating Activities with Engagement

In the Best Friends™ approach to dementia care, activities are all about relationships. What is friendship but doing things—playing together, working together, and being together? Friends might enjoy a spontaneous dinner or movie together, a regular workout at the gym or an evening yoga class, an outdoor adventure to the Grand Canyon or an indoor adventure to Las Vegas. Friends might get together with their families, gather for an event with their faith community, or walk or run to support a local charity.

Sharing meaningful activities bring friends closer together. Closeness and meaning are important for persons with dementia, who struggle to stay in the flow of life and are in danger of being cut off from others. That's why Virginia Bell calls shared activities "the art of being together."

Besides keeping people grounded in essential relationships, activities with engagement, whether planned or spontaneous, also help support a high quality of life for a person with dementia by:

- supporting a therapeutic environment that is rich in life-affirming moments
- building purpose and self-esteem
- helping people experience success
- keeping people physically active, which contributes to fall prevention and overall well-being

• fighting the boredom that can lead to behavior challenges and exit-seeking

Whatever your formal job description, when you are part of a Best Friends community or program, the role you play in activities is important. All of us should be engaged in formal, scheduled activities and informal in-between moments that build connection and relationship.

The Purpose of Activities

People do things for a reason. All of us have basic needs that are fulfilled by meaningful activities. In dementia care, activities are particularly important because they keep the person engaged in life, build self-esteem, fight depression, and promote physical fitness.

When we were preparing Volume 2 of *The Best Friend's Book of Alzheimer's Activities,* we asked 21 persons with early-stage dementia about what they wanted from activities. They told us very clearly how much they wanted to maintain a sense of purpose and productivity and that they still had something to contribute. In activities, they wanted to:

• enjoy time with friends and family

• advocate for themselves and others with dementia

• continue to help others as long as they could

• stay productive with volunteer work, chores, or meaningful activity

• embrace their creativity by doing photography, painting, writing, or being involved in music and the arts

• use the Internet to stay connected with their community and friends

• spend time in nature, in part because they were now seeing things they hadn't ever noticed or appreciated before

What other purposes draw us into activities? Let's look more closely.

Helping People to Be Productive or to Contribute

Most of us have a need to feel that our lives make a difference to someone or to a community. Maybe we are good at our jobs, volunteer in a children's charity, are good parents, or are good friends to others. Persons with dementia have reminded us that they also retain a need to be needed, to feel a part of the world, and to be productive (making dog biscuits for pets or creating gifts for children).

Helping People Experience Successes

Activities can lead to big and small successes. Children take pride in assembling their first model. A couple who together plant a beautiful garden can be proud of their accomplishment and enjoy the compliments that come from neighbors. Persons with dementia have faced many losses. Activities such as completing a word puzzle or a trivia game can help them enjoy new successes.

Helping People Play

Even though most of us work hard, having fun is still an important part of life. Skipping recreational or fun activities means missing out on one of life's joys. Persons with dementia often retain the ability to enjoy playing, to "lighten up" on life, tease, joke, and engage in activities, such as flying a kite, dancing, or enjoying a trip to the zoo. One purpose of activities is to have fun.

Helping People Be with Others

We participate in activities to be with friends, to meet new people, to be part of a club, or simply to feel like a part of society. People also benefit from socialization, including time spent reminiscing, attending a meeting of the Men's Club, or enjoying the sights of colorful costumes, the smell of food cooking, and the sounds of enjoyable music at a street fair.

Helping People Build Skills

We take part in society and do things to practice what we do well, sharpen old skills, or develop new ones. For example, a person can join the Toastmasters club to practice and improve public speaking skills. Persons with dementia may not necessarily be developing new skills, but activities such as participating in a simple bell choir or writing a group poem can help renew old skills and practice and preserve remaining ones.

Helping People Have a Sense of Control

All of us hope to have some control over our lives. Appropriate activities can help persons with dementia feel empowered and in charge of their world. Having a say in activities is one way to help them feel a sense of control. A resident in assisted living or skilled nursing might enjoy organizing supplies for an upcoming activity or serving on a building committee.

Helping People Feel Safe and Secure

All of us have a need for safety and security. If we live in a dangerous neighborhood, fear losing our jobs, or worry about money, these concerns can create stress and strain. Persons with dementia also can be prone to worry and fear. Dementia can be accompanied by confusion about time and place, or troubling delusions. Playing with pets, singing familiar songs, and looking at a book of family pictures can help recall warm feelings associated with past good times and help create the feeling that all is well.

Helping People Fill a Religious or Spiritual Need

Although not everyone professes a religious faith, we believe that everyone has a spiritual life. People have religious or spiritual needs that can be fulfilled by attending religious services, praying, singing or listening to old spiritual songs or hymns, writing poetry, creating art, walking in a forest, or showing compassion for others.

Helping People Experience Growth and Learning

Sometimes we take part in activities to learn more about a particular subject or for human growth. Persons with dementia may or may not be able to learn new information, but they still can enjoy the experience of being presented interesting new material. Satisfaction and pleasure come from participation in a learning situation, like the simple class on the famous Golden Gate Bridge in the sidebar.

Why Not Teach a Class on the Golden Gate Bridge?

- Use the Internet to learn all you can about San Francisco's world famous Golden Gate Bridge.
- Discuss the history of the bridge and show old pictures of its construction.
- Share stories about visiting San Francisco.
- Serve San Francisco–style sourdough bread.
- Paint pictures of the bridge and debate the exact color of its "gold."
- Have fun making Rice-A-Roni, advertised as the "San Francisco Treat®" (even though it isn't from San Francisco).
- Discuss the city's role in the 1960s hippie movement.
- Sing the famous song "I Left My Heart in San Francisco."

Activities versus Engagement

Whether you work in a home setting, a day program, or residential care, doing things with a person with dementia is probably part of your job. Your job could include chores for the person in home, leading a music program at a day center, calling bingo, or leading an exercise class in a residential care community. You may be an administrator who cooks an occasional Sunday pancake breakfast for your residents or an occupational therapist who periodically brings your dog to work to visit with clients.

All of these activities are worthwhile, and in many settings they are listed on an activity calendar. But a Best Friends care partner knows that the calendar is just the beginning. An ordinary activity can be turned into something more meaningful!

Let's tackle bingo. Using what we call *engagement,* this simple game can become a window into something more meaningful: a chance to talk and connect, share Life Stories, offer opinions, and develop more closeness. Bingo can provide opportunities for:

- sharing stories during a break
- introducing participants to each other with some interesting Life Story trivia
- listening to some music before and after
- sitting next to a Best Friend who helps you play the game, perhaps giving you a few hugs along the way when you win

Simply put, bingo is an activity, and if you just call the numbers and work your way through the game, you've had some fun and checked the activity off your list. If you think about making the most of some of the in-between moments of the game, you've now achieved engagement, an opportunity to have more meaningful, one-on-one moments between friends that builds a feeling of connection and intimacy.

Our two volumes of *The Best Friends Book of Alzheimer's Activities* show how more than 300 activities can be done with engagement. Each one offers basic directions for the activity (instructions, supplies, variations) and a section called "The Best Friends Way," which offers ideas and options that foster one-on-one engagement. Figure 6.1 shows how an ordinary activity such as doing laundry can be done with engagement. For example, instead of simply folding towels, a Best Friends care partner can reminisce about old ways of doing laundry, talk about favorite colors of clothes, or joke about laundry mishaps.

LAUNDRY: The Basics ―――――――――――――

There are a surprising number of steps to doing the laundry, including gathering clothes to be washed, sorting clothes, putting clothes in the washer, adding detergent, transferring clothes to the dryer, hanging clothes outside to dry, folding, pressing, ironing, and putting clothes away. Some garments require hand washing.

Try to figure out the most appropriate step or steps for the *person*. Let that be the *person's* specific job. Talk about his or her help in keeping the laundry caught up and how much you appreciate the contribution.

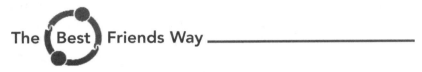

The (Best) Friends Way ――――――――――――

Life Story: Many *persons* have been in charge of the laundry all of their lives. Does the *person* seem to have an interest in helping with the laundry now? Did he or she ever work in a laundry or help other individuals with their laundry?

Humor: Laugh together about the time you washed a red sock with all the whites and turned everything pink! Or comment that there are ten socks without a matching one; the washer must be eating the socks!

Early Dementia: *Persons* may be completely functional in a task as familiar as operating the washer and dryer. They may take great pride in washing by hand some of their articles of clothing.

Late Dementia: *Persons* can find meaning in folding clothes, especially bath towels, tea towels, and napkins.

Old Sayings: "Starched stiff enough to stand alone."

Old Skills: Folding, ironing, and hanging clothes out to dry are activities many people conducted all of their lives.

Sensory: The soft feel of fabric and the clean smell of clothes can be wonderfully refreshing. And if hanging clothes outside is the order of the day, the whole outside is a sensory show.

Conversation: Reminisce, "Do you remember your mother using a washboard to clean the clothes?" "Did you hang your clothes out to dry on a line?" Ask for advice, "What is the best way to get out a stain?" Compliment, "Marilyn, you must have worked so hard to send your girls to school in a clean starched dress every day" or "Matt, I can tell you learned how to iron in the Marines. I've never seen neater pants with such a crisp look."

Figure 6.1. Laundry activity. (Reprinted from Bell & Troxel, *The Best Friend's Book of Alzheimer's Activities, Volume One*).

Take the outdoor walk. Exercise is essential; walking, no matter what, is good. But if during the walk we take the time to stop and notice a flower or a hummingbird, reminisce about making daisy chains, or point out favorite colors, then we are turning a simple activity into a major opportunity for engagement.

Almost everything can become an extended, interesting opportunity for engagement. A simple handshake can lead to a discussion about fingernail polish, gloves, work done by hand, "lifelines," rings on fingers, promise rings, weddings, and more. A teapot can be enjoyed for its beauty, and discussions can follow about making tea, reading tea leaves, the different flavors of tea, and the Boston Tea Party.

Because the bottom line of the Best Friends approach is to focus on the person rather than the task, the main lens the Best Friends care partner brings to activities is keeping the focus on the process, not the result. Virginia Bell has really been ahead of her time on this topic. For years, she has advocated for unstructured, spontaneous activities because she has seen their power in action at the Best Friends™ Day Center. To her, it's the in-between moments, particularly ones that draw on information and values from the Life Story, that let us practice the art of being together. Thus, a Best Friends program should have an innovative, fun-filled calendar *and* team members who engage in small talk, offer welcomed hugs, join people in spontaneous walks, or take time to discuss a favorite recipe.

In a good dementia program, all of the bases are covered: structured moments, spontaneous moments, group activities, and time spent one-on-one. Use the Best Friends approach to support an activity and engagement program that is full of life and makes the most of the moments between "official" activities, when we can really step up and be a Best Friends care partner to a friend with dementia.

Activities Done the Best Friends Way

For Best Friends care partners, the following concepts are essential to creating a successful activity program that engages the person, and hopefully engages you and your team, too!

The art of activities is not in what is done; it is in the doing. The *process* of the activity is always more important than the *result* or end product. If folding towels is accompanied by smiles, conversation, friendly gossip, discussion about fabrics and colors, and praise for a job well done, it should not matter if the towels are not folded with perfect edges. If you are putting together kits

The Best Friends Approach to Activities

- The art of activities isn't in what's done; it's in the doing.
- Activities often need to be initiated by a Best Friends care partner.
- Activities should be individualized and should tap into past interests and skills.
- Activities should be adult in nature.
- Activities should stimulate the five senses (hearing, sight, smell, taste, and touch).
- Activities should tap into remaining physical skills.
- Activities should fulfill spiritual and/or religious needs.
- Activities should recall the work-related past.
- Personal care is an activity, not just a task.
- Doing nothing is actually doing something.
- Activities should be voluntary.
- Intergenerational activities are especially desirable.
- Activities can be short.
- Activities we think will never work sometimes do.

to make bird feeders, take time to discuss the miracles of nature, humming-birds, and the importance of giving our "feathered friends" some good food throughout winter. It doesn't matter if the feeder isn't perfectly painted.

Activities often need to be initiated by a Best Friends care partner. Persons with dementia sometimes lose the ability to initiate activities. A retired painter, for example, may still enjoy painting, but he may have to be handed the brush and cued about how to dip the brush in paint and stroke the canvas. Often, extra encouragement is all that is needed to conduct a successful activity: "Mike, I'm playing softball this weekend. Would you help me warm up?" (and then having a fun game of catch). If the answer is no, remember not to give up the first time; keep trying to turn that *no* into a *yes*. Take special note of our use of the word "often" in this paragraph. We *often* have to initiate but not *always*. Persons may often take your hand to suggest a walk, give you a hug out of the blue, or even take down a puzzle from a shelf and begin working on it, waiting for a Best Friend to help.

Activities should be voluntary. Like the rest of us, most persons with dementia will not do something they do not enjoy or find satisfying.

No one should be forced to do something against his or her will, particularly in the realm of activities. But there are certainly ways you can encourage participation. For example, some care partners have found that if they begin an activity in front of the person, he or she may become interested and then take over the task and continue working happily for a period of time. Another good idea is to build some "anchors" into your day, such as exercise at 11 a.m. and music after dinner. The person (or people in a group setting) may begin to associate that time of day with the activity, encouraging attendance.

Activities should be individualized and should tap into past interests and skills. The Life Story should be mined for ideas about activities. A person who enjoyed playing cards, for example, might not be able to play poker or bridge anymore but might enjoy playing a simpler game with assistance, such as shuffling the deck, checking the deck to find missing cards, or simply being present and watching others play. A retired English teacher may enjoy reading Emily Dickinson's poetry. A woman who loved to play the piano may still enjoy being prompted to play a simple old tune.

Sometimes persons with dementia may realize their losses and not want to do something they used to do quite well. It's always okay to try, but if the person doesn't want to paint (even if he was once a masterful painter), respect his preference.

Activities should be adult in nature. Activities that are unnecessarily juvenile can provoke annoyance or lead to lack of participation. Some respond to dolls or children's toys, but there is no reason to keep *all* activities at this level. We generally frown on using childlike objects or materials, such as crayons, in memory care programs, unless, for example, a former kindergarten teacher enjoys using crayons because they are tied into her past work. Another possible exception could be adults who are willing to participate in childlike activities when working alongside children or making something for children, such as a gift for a grandchild.

Activities stimulate the five senses (hearing, sight, smell, taste, touch). Although some senses are diminished by age, many remain strong. The most successful activities stimulate more than one sense. Gardening, for example, involves touching wet soil, smelling different flowers, hearing the sound of footsteps on autumn leaves, tasting fruit from a tree or a tomato from a vine, and seeing vivid colors in a variety of plants. Almost any activity can be expanded to facilitate a more sensory experience. When discussing old cars, you might weave in music featuring automobiles (dozens of examples can be found on the Internet), pass around an old-fashioned chamois cloth to feel, or take the guys outside and wash a car!

Activities tap into remaining physical skills. Many persons with dementia remain in remarkably good physical condition, including having good hand–eye coordination. Activities should take advantage of remaining skills by including exercise, walking, active chores, or other physical tasks and games. There is evidence that regular exercise may delay the onset of Alzheimer's disease until later in life and that exercise may slow decline in those who already have dementia. Exercise also builds strength and can prevent falls.

Activities recall the work-related past. Many persons with dementia enjoy activities that touch on their work-related past, in part because work played an enormous role in their lives. A librarian may want to organize a shelf of books. A homemaker may enjoy organizational tasks or a discussion about canning fruits and vegetables. This seems particularly true for men, who are generally harder to engage. The guys in your program may enjoy tasks such as adding up numbers (former accountant), giving educational advice (former school principal), helping plan an outing (business owner or manager), or taking on a simple carpentry project (someone who worked with his hands).

Personal care is an activity, more than a task. One of our favorite writers on dementia care, occupational therapist Jitka Zgola, talks about the importance of reframing ADLs or personal care into an activity in her book *Care That Works: A Relationship Approach to Persons with Dementia* (1999). One funny example Jitka shares is about an aide who when giving a bath to a woman in memory care says, "Let's hurry up, the aromatherapy class is about to begin!" (p. 169). She points out the absurdity of leaving behind a bath that already *is* satisfying to the body, senses, and soul. Take time when doing personal care to reminisce, talk about the colors of the clothes or the shade of lipstick, or comment on the scented soap. This adds great value to the experience and fosters cooperation instead of struggle. The sidebar "Get Your Exercise!" shares more ideas for turning personal care into an activity.

Doing nothing is actually doing something. Even good friends enjoy quiet times together, perhaps just sitting in the living room listening to music or watching the world go by through a picture window. Sometimes the person is content just to be present, observing others at work, or, depending on his or her level of dementia, the person may simply enjoy time alone. Many in-home workers take time to sit outside in the backyard or front porch with the person, a simple, pleasant activity that helps the person take in lots of sensory stimulation while enjoying the sights and sounds of the neighborhood.

Intergenerational activities are especially desirable. Any staff member of an adult day center with links to a child care center can testify to the fact that intergenerational activities are extremely successful. Both generations benefit from the exchange, and many persons with dementia enjoy being able to help young people complete a task or project. Again, individual differences must be recognized; not everyone loves kids and pets.

Activities can be short. Sometimes the person's attention span makes an extended activity difficult. Even very brief activities, repeated often, can fill a day—taking a short walk, singing a favorite song, organizing a drawer of socks or scarves, sorting poker chips, or dusting a table. See our list of "30 Activities to Do in 30 Seconds or Less" in the sidebar.

Activities we think will never work sometimes do. Many families respond to an activity calendar by saying "my loved one would never do a country-western line dance." We have found that the opposite is true. Persons with dementia sometimes surprise us with their willingness to try something new, particularly if they feel safe in their environment and are surrounded by caring staff. Rather than thinking about the pros and cons of an invitation to do something (do we really want to go to the beach on the weekend, when it will be crowded?), they may be making their decisions more "in the moment" or based upon how our staff as Best Friends have made them feel (if staff show enthusiasm going on an outing to the beach).

Getting Started
Putting Your Knack to Work

We've looked at the *why* of creative, low-cost activities. The *how* comes from you! Put your Knack to work. Get inspired by a person's home. Chat on the patio about hummingbirds, blooming flowers, or overdue fence repairs. Draw on your own hobbies, talents, and interests. If you love scrapbooking, create scrapbooks together. If you enjoy baking, spend some time making cupcakes with residents. If you are interested in history, talk with your in-home client about his early years building bridges or working in Alaska.

Relying on your own inspiration and your growing skills as a Best Friends care partner, you can use the following ideas as a springboard for dozens more ideas you can customize to the needs and wishes of your Best Friends.

Doing Chores

Even in late-stage dementia, chores can help people feel the satisfaction they felt during their working lives. Ask the person to help. "Lester, could you help me plant these tulips? You've got such a special touch with plants." Asking the question helps initiate the task and praises the person's skills. Afterward, give a compliment. "Thanks to you, we'll have a beautiful garden in the spring." Remember to make room for spontaneous moments of fun, like squirting each other with a hose!

- Gardening involves many senses and can evoke a person's pride in the gardens created and maintained.
- Polishing the furniture or straightening art around the home can make the person feel useful.
- Folding clothes can keep hand–eye coordination intact.
- Drying dishes can evoke early family memories.
- Raking leaves or sweeping a porch can be good exercise.
- Stirring a pot can be a chance to smell strong spices.
- Organizing a box of supplies, handing out music programs, or helping the maintenance guy make his rounds can make a person feel needed and appreciated.

Enjoying Animals and Pets

Pets can provide unconditional love. In home settings, pets can provide the person with a sense of responsibility and pride about participating in the care of an animal, even if it's just helping feed the cat or fish. In a dementia program, consider adopting a cat or dog or making a connection to the many formal and informal pet therapy programs. If that's not possible, consider shelling peanuts for the neighborhood squirrels or making a group project of maintaining your bird feeders. Even persons in late-stage dementia can enjoy these activities:

- Listening to a bird sing can be an impromptu concert.
- Baking dog biscuits for your adopted dog or pet rescue program (or to distribute to visiting or resident pets) can add a welcome sense of purpose. Consider setting an annual goal for the number of dog biscuits you will make or selling them as a fundraiser for the local Alzheimer's association or society.

Making the Most of Music

Music and song lyrics survive in the brain of persons with dementia longer than words and language. This is why so many people recall the lyrics of old songs and enjoy singing and music. Most programs take advantage of music's magic, but we find they could do more. Consider these:

- Scheduling an evening concert can engage senses and end the day with a calm, peaceful feeling.
- Singing along to old movie musicals with subtitles can be an opportunity for a visiting family member to enjoy some simple time with her mom or dad.
- Humming or singing a resident's favorite song can reduce anxiety.
- Creating a "signature song" for a particular activity—like playing old-fashioned marching band music before every exercise—can encourage a resident to leave his room and walk down the hall to the class.
- Dancing can be good fun any time!

Celebrating Food and Dining

Food and dining are pleasures most of us look forward to every day. Does your dining program create a warm and festive atmosphere? Have you checked the Life Story to discover each person's food preferences? Is there conversation over the meal? Baking and cooking remain great activity ideas. Ask for some family recipes. If you have a resident from Italy, bake her favorite lasagna or Italian cookie. The excellent program Dining with Friends, from the Alzheimer's Resource Center of Connecticut, uses principles around the acronym DINE (Dining is social: Independence, Nutrition, and Environment) to help you create a lovely, social, and respectful dining experience for people with dementia. (See the Suggested Resources.)

30 Activities to Do in 30 Seconds or Less

- Greet the person by name.
- Make eye contact and smile.
- Shake hands.
- Ask someone to "show me" an object.
- Gently tease: "Mr. Smith, I just saw you eat dessert first!"
- Tell someone he or she is loved.
- Give a sustained bear hug.
- Give a compliment: "Wow! You're looking pretty spiffy today, Margie."
- Ask an open-ended question: "How are you feeling today, Mike?"
- Ask an opinion: "What do you think of my new necktie? Does it match my shirt?"
- Play a quick game of catch.
- Notice an unusual bird outside the window.
- Evoke a memory from the person's Life Story: "Tell me about that grandfather of yours who was a country doctor. Did he really make house calls?"
- Give a hand massage.
- Share a new hand lotion and talk about its pleasant scent.
- Blow bubbles.
- Slip a little treat to someone (be certain it's dietetically okay).
- Share a magic trick.
- Show off family photos of a new grandchild.
- Blow up a balloon and bat it around.
- Look at a flower arrangement and compare colors, textures, and scents.
- Ask for advice on a recipe.
- Tell a funny story or two.
- Do a quick dance to some fun music playing in the background.
- Notice vivid colors in an unusual dress or shirt.
- Ask for help with a chore, such as folding a towel, helping make a bed, or squirting some wax onto a piece of furniture to be polished.
- Try on a hat or hats.
- Try on a new shade of lipstick.
- Clown around for a moment, making funny faces, or throwing your hands in the air and spinning around once or twice in a silly dance.
- Step outdoors for some fresh air.

Get Your Exercise!

Exercise classes are a great way to help persons with dementia benefit their brains and bodies by exercising twice a day. Consider:

- chair exercises, dance, or yoga
- T'ai chi (can be modified for chairs)
- walking inside or outside
- simple stretching or stretching with Therabands™ (stretchy fabric that comes in a variety of strengths)
- ball tosses
- playing parachutes, where everyone holds part of a big fabric parachute and a ball is put in the middle and bounced around
- conducting music with chopsticks
- using simple weights
- going to a gym or using exercise equipment with supervision from staff

Ask a physical therapist to do some individual assessments and coaching along with some general support for your program. To find a fitness professional who specializes in long-term care, including dementia care, check the International Council on Active Aging (www.icaa.cc).

Performing Personal Care

Best Friends care partners with Knack can turn the sometimes daunting tasks of personal care into activities:

- Taking a bath can become a bubble bath, with laughter and bubble blowing.
- Dressing can become a fashion show.
- Brushing teeth can become a taste test for a new toothpaste.
- Combing hair can become an opportunity for a quiet sing-along.
- Toileting can be a time to provide extra reassurance.
- Applying makeup can be a time to make fun faces in the mirror.
- Giving a manicure can be a time to compliment the person.
- Eating a meal can be a time to ask for an opinion.

Some food-related activities include:

- An ice cream cone or ice cream social can evoke happy childhood memories.
- Making a pie from scratch allows opportunity for conversation and advice ("How do you make a good crust?").
- Food preferences can lead to laughter, as groups discuss who enjoys hot and spicy food or who must have chocolate every day.
- Cookbooks can be reviewed to plan a dinner party menu, helping a person feel productive.
- Setting a table can be an opportunity for the person to feel successful.

Playing Word Games

Vocabulary learned long ago can be retrieved through clever word games. These activities tend to work well in group settings or as part of a small family gathering. Besides evoking long car drives or family vacations, these games are successful because everyone in the room can participate. Because many word games are open-ended, there are almost unlimited right answers. The following ideas for word games can be useful:

- Naming opposites, such as up and down, top and bottom, and right and left, can easily be played at a doctor's office, during a trip, or during other potentially stressful times.
- Listing every word with a certain color, such as Red Sea, red sky, red flag, red-handed, and redhead, can allow people to participate in group activities.
- Composing a get-well card together can fulfill the need to help others.
- Using Scrabble letters to spell out key words from the person's past can be a way to honor his or her Life Story and touch on past achievements.
- Naming state capitals can be a pleasurable brain fitness game in a day center.

Enjoying Time with Children

Children can be especially loving and accepting of people with dementia. Besides bringing joy and offering opportunities to help or teach young people, intergenerational activities can also be valuable to children with no nearby grandparents. The possibilities are endless for active (tossing a ball, painting a picture) or passive (listening to music, hearing someone read poems) experiences:

- Making a Halloween mask together can involve both individuals in a fulfilling art project.
- Reading stories aloud to one another can be an opportunity for praise.
- Walking together can provide exercise and a chance to pick wildflowers.
- Enjoying the festivities surrounding a common birthday (blowing out candles, exchanging presents, singing "Happy Birthday," and eating birthday cake) can evoke smiles and laughter.
- Being with children can make it acceptable for adults to play child-like games and work simple puzzles.
- Working on the computer together can help build bonds as you help the person have a video chat with family members or play simple games.

Savoring Quiet Time

Setting aside time for quiet reflection or watching the world go by can calm the person and help care partners recharge their batteries. Often, this quiet time can be achieved by identifying daily rituals the person has previously enjoyed. The following activities provide quiet moments:

- Visiting the library to flip through the latest magazines in a quiet, studious atmosphere can often be calming to the person.
- Starting a new tradition of afternoon "high tea" and cookies can build a daily ritual.
- Taking a daily walk focuses the person on a single task and can be equally enjoyed by the care partner.
- Watching hummingbirds sip nectar from flowers can help the person connect with nature.

Honoring Spiritual Traditions

The Dementia Bill of Rights affirms the right to be with individuals who know one's Life Story, including cultural and spiritual traditions. The Life Story can give you clues on how to touch and nurture the person's spirit until the very end. The following activities can fulfill the person's spiritual needs:

- Reading aloud from the Bible or other religious texts can be reassuring.
- Listening to organ music or gospel music can evoke past memories of church activities.
- Praying remains a powerful, symbolic act for many people.
- Celebrating religious holidays can help a person feel connected.
- Involving the person in helping a local charity can help him or her feel compassion for others.
- Continuing to attend religious services can help a person feel valued.
- Seeing a beautiful sunrise can lift a person's spirit and make him or her feel more attuned to the universe.

Exploring the Artistic Self

Daphne Gormley of Santa Barbara, a person with younger-onset dementia who was featured in Maria Shriver's 2009 HBO special "The Alzheimer's Project," was also a friend of Virginia Bell and David Troxel. After her diagnosis, when she was no longer able to work as an astrophysicist

Doing Activities that Benefit People at Different Stages of Dementia

How can you design activities that meet the needs of persons who are at different stages of dementia or who have differing (remaining) skills and abilities—especially if staffing challenges make it difficult to provide parallel programming?

One answer is to look for programs and activities that appeal to a wide range of people. Spending time outdoors is a group activity that appeals to almost everyone. So are music and exercise. It's perfectly fine if some residents do all of the stretches and movements while others do one or two, because all residents are active and enjoying the group activity. Music is therapeutic, whether someone is singing or listening quietly on the sidelines. Another favorite "multistage" activity is collage. Some persons with dementia can help plan the topic or organize the supplies. Some can cut out fabric, draw, paint, or help assemble and apply glue. Others may be able to press down on the fabric. Late in dementia they can enjoy touching the collage and its various components or simply enjoy the final piece of art.

(she had worked on NASA's Hubble space telescope), she turned to the arts and became an accomplished artist. She told everyone that art allowed her to focus on what she could still do instead of what she had lost. She found her art to be "joyful" and certainly therapeutic. Daphne died in 2012, but her colorful and fascinating artwork, included in David and Virginia's presentations throughout the world, has inspired many people to look at dementia in a new way.

"Arts and crafts provide a wonderful opportunity for people to utilize their remaining strengths and abilities," says Robin Hamon, co-author of both volumes of *The Best Friends Book of Alzheimer's Activities*. "The nonverbal language of art frees persons who have trouble with the complexity of language. Feelings that cannot be expressed in words can often be expressed in art. The sensory exploration of color and texture is stimulating and satisfying."

Persons with dementia may enjoy the following creative arts and crafts projects:

- drawing or painting a memory from childhood, such as a house, school, creek, or forest
- recognizing familiar paintings seen in an oversized art book
- using clay to sculpt an animal
- assembling a mobile from objects gathered on an impromptu scavenger hunt (pinecones, leaves, feathers)
- creating sun catchers for the windows
- filling oranges with dried cloves to give as gifts
- designing decorations for a holiday party

Conclusion

Imagine that you have moved your mother or grandmother into a residential care program, signed her up for a day center, or hired an in-home care partner. How would you feel if you saw Mom sleeping in her chair all day, sitting alone in front of the television, or coloring in a children's coloring book? How would you feel if activities stopped at 5 p.m. on weekdays and were nonexistent on weekends?

The opposite of this bleak picture is engagement, a hallmark of an outstanding dementia program. Engagement touches a person spiritually, builds relationships, fosters happiness, reduces challenging behaviors, and actually makes your job easier and more fulfilling. Creating a rich social atmosphere in which people are active and engaged throughout the day is good for anyone with dementia. It also creates a caring, interesting community environment—a good place to live and work.

It's no accident that many organizations are rethinking job titles in the area of dementia care. Instead of a director of activities, we have encountered a director of life engagement, director of enrichment, and in one case a director of fun! These titles underlie a growing movement to build more life into our programs and break away from some of the bad habits of the past. Implementing the ideas in this chapter will help support this movement and acknowledge that we are all enriched by the Best Friends approach.

CHAPTER 7

Best Friends and Behavior That Is Challenging for Staff

"Why do persons with dementia have good days and bad days?" we were once asked. Our response was, "Don't we *all* have good days and bad days?"

With the Best Friends™ approach, there will be lots of good days. Knowing and using the Life Story, keeping the person engaged in creative programs, communicating well, and using Knack all bring out the best in someone with dementia. Of course, challenges inevitably arise, as confusion, lack of judgment, personality changes, and cognitive decline all accompany dementia. This chapter focuses on those tougher times.

What do you do as Best Friends staff when the person is angry, agitated, deeply confused, distrustful, suspicious, sad or withdrawn, or wanting to walk out the front door on a bitter cold night in pajamas? How do you handle upsetting sexual behavior, even while knowing that sexuality is part of life? How do you deal with a person who simply says no to just about everything?

In some care settings, behavior is "treated" with psychotropic medications, which may help when the person exhibits dangerous, distrustful, suspicious, aggressive, or antisocial behaviors that scare staff and family. The problem is that these medications can have highly variable efficacy, often make matters worse, and have troubling side effects. Sedating a person may diminish or suppress a behavior but also may trigger new challenges, such as lethargy (which can contribute to skin

129

problems and urinary tract infections) or increased confusion (which damages quality of life). There is also a greater risk of falls, which can be devastating to people who may already be frail.

The Dementia Bill of Rights reflects our point of view very clearly in stating that persons with dementia have the right to be free from psychotropic medications whenever possible. A sedated life is not a good life. Hugs are better than drugs!

Let's see how the Best Friends approach can inspire you to address behavior challenges with confidence and success.

Empathy Is the Key

For Best Friends care partners, empathy is essential. We must "walk a mile in the shoes" of the person with memory loss and confusion. Rebecca Riley helped us walk that mile by describing her experience of dementia in her diary:

- *Depression*
- *Can't say what I want.*
- *Afraid I can't express my thoughts and words—thus I remain silent and become depressed.*
- *I need conversation to be slowly.*
- *It is difficult to follow conversation with so much noise.*
- *I feel that people turn me off because I cannot express myself.*
- *I dislike social workers, nurses, and friends who do not treat me as a real person.*
- *It is difficult to live one day at a time.*

Rebecca's words help us to understand that persons with dementia have all of the same feelings as the rest of us. Rebecca felt some fear and frustration. She could sense when those around her weren't treating her with respect. One can imagine Rebecca becoming angry if she had been placed in a situation where she had lost control of her life and was surrounded by staff who were not supportive or tuned in to her needs, especially as her ability to articulate those needs declined.

Empathy is also important because persons with dementia like Rebecca can be less resilient to illness and emotional upset than the rest of us. You and I may be able to shake off a headache ("I've taken the aspirin. I'll feel better soon"), but pain seems to hit persons with dementia especially hard and can be a root cause of behavior challenges. You and I may worry (flight turbulence), but we can process that worry ("We are flying through strong winds"), we can think about it ("We will soon be through this rough patch of air"), and we can calm ourselves ("I'll keep reading my book until we land"). You may find in persons with dementia that a minor worry left unattended blows up into a full-scale anxiety attack ("When is my ride coming?" "Did I miss that appointment?").

Our experience has taught us that having dementia is like taking a trip to a foreign country where customs are different, the currency is unfamiliar, and you don't speak the language. For Irene Hong, a volunteer at the Best Friends™ Day Center, traveling to Taiwan to visit her grandmother confirmed this truth!

Empathy can also help us reinterpret behaviors that seem strange, unusual, or upsetting as the person's way of coping with the experience of dementia. Hiding a purse or wallet is a normal action any of us would take if we believed someone was trying to steal our valuables. Most of us might become a bit suspicious if we thought others were talking about us behind our backs or asking us to do something we don't understand.

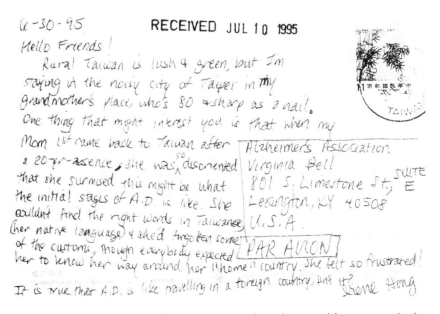

Figure 7.1.   Postcard from student Irene Hong, who volunteered for one year in the Helping Hand of Lexington, Kentucky.

Coming to the United States

Many staff in long-term care have emigrated to the United States from other countries. A good empathy-building exercise is to ask your memory care team to describe their first days in the United States. These staff members may describe their harrowing first trip on a freeway, their struggles to learn English and handle money, or their first time navigating a big grocery store. Make the point that their stress and fear were perfectly normal, as are the emotions of people with dementia. End the discussion on a high note. Ask who recalls someone who was particularly kind or helpful during those first days—perhaps a friendly store clerk or neighbor. How did that feel? Remind staff that we want to be a friendly face and supporter of the person with dementia. The sharing of similar experiences helps staff develop empathy.

Creative Problem Solving to Address Behaviors in Dementia

The Best Friends approach to creatively address behaviors in dementia has three steps.

First, Best Friends staff look carefully at what might be triggering a behavior: the environment, illness, medication issues, or any unmet needs. This is especially important as dementia progresses. Early on, a person can communicate feelings and challenges using words. Later on, his or her behaviors articulate what words cannot. Pain may be expressed by yelling or striking out, boredom by walking out of the house unaccompanied, and loneliness by tears. Sometimes just "diagnosing" the behavior is enough to address it, for example, by treating a toothache or giving a snack to a person who is hungry. It's your job to stay alert and be a detective, looking for clues and cues when they come up.

Second, if the behavior continues, refer to and use the Life Story for insight and inspiration. You may discover a specific cause of behavior (your resident is not a morning person and a staff member tried to get him up and going too early), or else find great material to work with to move the person's emotions and behavior to a better place (ask the person to show you her favorite scrapbooks of her family).

Third, be sure to communicate your best ideas to each other. Sometimes one shift in residential care is doing well but another shift is not. Get your team together to brainstorm approaches and share best practices. For example, if the morning shift has discovered that smaller portions on the plate actually encourage the resident to eat a full break- fast, be sure that the evening shift knows this for dinner. Encouraging group problem solving and brainstorming respects the talents of your Best Friends team and can lead to some very creative solutions.

On the second page of the comic strip that follows, see how Paulina and her team, whom we first met in the comic strip in Chapter 2, use the following three steps to resolve a challenge around helping Joe with bathing.

Step One: Diagnosing Behavior

To determine what is triggering the behavior,

- Stop, look, and listen.
- Rule out illness and medication issues.
- Look for an unmet need.
- Check the environment.

Stop, Look, and Listen

Behavior is nearly always responsive. When a behavior happens, take a moment to assess the situation and look for causes or triggers. Ask if this is a long-standing issue (worry about getting picked up from the day center at the end of the day) or something new (a visit from grand- children who are too loud). Sometimes taking a good step back will provide some clues and cues (maybe the person was especially fatigued after an outing or staff rushed him or her).

Rule Out Illness and Medication Issues

Be particularly vigilant for sudden changes in behavior. Alzheimer's dis- ease and other dementias tend to be slow and progressive. If you have a normally happy, easygoing person who suddenly seems upset, agitated, or withdrawn, it's usually a sign of pain or illness (often the notoriously behavior-changing urinary tract infection).

Pain can come on quickly (muscle pain or a toothache) or be pres- ent over time with chronic illness (arthritis). It's important to be sure that your program takes steps to identify and manage pain, because pain can damage quality of life and cause behavior challenges. Similarly, depression often goes untreated in persons with dementia. The use of antidepressant medications combined with increased attention and activity can help manage this challenge. Treating depression improves quality of life.

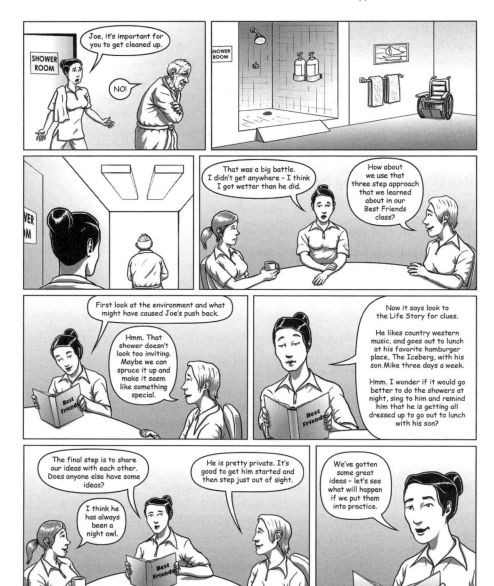

Figure 7.2.

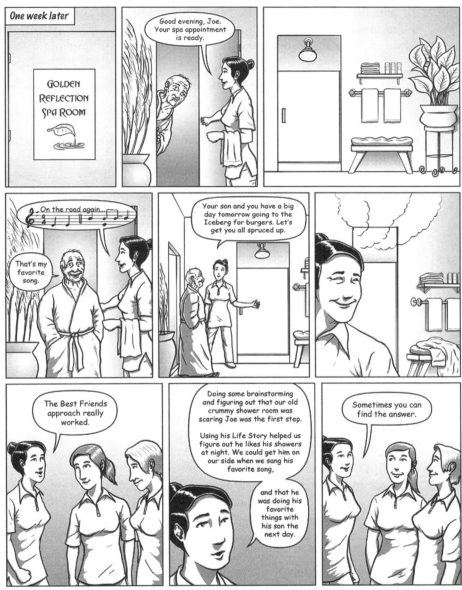

Figure 7.2. *(continued)*

Finally, it's always important to look at the medications a person is taking, including over-the-counter medications. Could the person be taking pills in the wrong amounts, at the wrong times, or not at all? Could one prescription be reacting with another? Evaluate the situation with a good pharmacist.

Look for An Unmet Need

Sometimes we can find a simple answer for a person's behavior. Was the person hungry, or did he or she have to go the bathroom? Was it an emotional need the person was trying to express? Perhaps the person was lonely or sad, and that triggered a behavior. As discussed in Chapter 6, boredom can be an enemy for a person with dementia. Are we doing all we can to engage him or her in meaningful activity that builds feelings of self-esteem and success? The bottom line is that behavior often communicates a message. When you figure out what the unmet need is, you move toward a solution.

Check the Environment

Is the environment contributing to some kind of responsive behavior? Persons with dementia can be very sensitive to noise, glare from a window (can actually be painful to an older adult's eye), or other stimuli from the environment. Older adults are also susceptible to deficits in the environment, especially poor lighting. In fact, shadows and dim lights increase fall risks. Simple environmental designs can make a difference. For example, a person who is urinating on the floor of the bathroom may not be able to differentiate a white toilet seat from the white ceramic bowl. White floors and white walls only make it harder. Adding contrasting flooring or wall color and a colored toilet lid might solve this bathroom problem right away.

Examining the environment is especially important for Best Friends care partners who provide in-home care. David Troxel once worked with a couple in their 80s who were living in their home. When the wife, who had Alzheimer's, started expressing significant suspicions about her husband, David suspected that their dark, poorly lit, and cluttered home might be contributing to her expressions of distrust and suspicion. After conferring with David, the couple's son took steps to improve the lighting and clean up the house. He instructed his dad to open the curtains and turn on the lights late in the day and into the evening.

David's hunch paid off. Her distrust and suspicions *were* being fueled by her poor vision coupled with terrible lighting. Adding some light and sunshine and cleaning up the house saved the day, and her suspicions diminished significantly. This "treatment" was vastly more effective than treating her with psychotropic medications, which could have diminished her quality of life and not fixed the problem, because the poor lighting and cluttered house would have remained triggers for her suspicions.

Step Two: Mine the Life Story for Ideas About Behavior

The Life Story holds a wealth of information that can be used to address behavior challenges. A Life Story can:

- help you to know favorite stories or happy experiences to mention
- help you understand the person's personality
- inform you about topics to avoid
- inspire activities that help the person find purpose and meaning
- offer key information to help you more skillfully redirect the person when needed.

A Life Story can help you to know favorite stories or happy experiences to mention.

Reviewing the person's Life Story may help you discover the one favorite subject that changes the mood from good to bad (discussing childhood trips to a baseball game or offering a favorite food). You may find out that the person previously acted in local theater companies and could ask him to do some "dramatic readings" that enhance his sense of belonging and bring a smile to his face.

A Life Story can help you understand the person's personality.

Has the person always been an ambitious, hardworking overachiever? Has he or she always been mellow and relaxed? Has your new resident always had a temper or been good natured? Knowing the person's past personality can be important as you organize your response to behavior. For example, if an in-home client yells at you a few times a day and you discover he has always been pretty challenging, it might help you to learn to simply roll with it and not take his outbursts too personally. If the person yelling at you is normally good natured, you may want to dig a bit deeper to understand the causes and try to address her unmet need.

Working with Rebecca, Virginia Bell understood that her personality involved being productive and purposeful. Therefore, Virginia tried to organize activities that would keep Rebecca busy and engaged, everything from reviewing paperwork at the day center to helping set up supplies for an activity.

A Life Story can inform you about topics to avoid.

The Life Story can help you to know what subjects to avoid or how to respond when they arise, including past trauma. Could behavior that is challenging to staff be triggered by memories of the Vietnam War while the person is watching a program on the History Channel, or by recalling during pet therapy a long-ago dog bite? Once you have this understanding, you may be able to prevent these challenges (e.g., not visiting an animal shelter or avoiding war movies). Knowing about past troubles can also help us respond more sensitively when unpleasant memories do arise (letting the person talk about his wartime experiences and offering supportive words ("It took a lot of courage to go through that time, Bob. You are a real hero.").

A Life Story can inspire activities that help the person find purpose and meaning.

The Life Story can suggest ways to engage the person in a meaningful task that can help him or her feel productive and needed. David has often described this concept as finding a "job" for the person: "So many elders have had productive and meaningful lives. Having purpose supports happiness and calm and lowers the chances of behavior that is challenging." With some humor, David notes that once a person accepts a role or job, he or she often holds on to it with great intensity. If a resident's job is to set out the menus, she may get quite upset if another resident tries to move in on her territory!

A Life Story can offer key information to help you more skillfully redirect the person when needed.

The classic way to manage behavior is to redirect:

• Listen to what the person is saying.

• Show empathy.

• Redirect by bringing up a favorite subject or key element from the Life Story.

• Offer a favorite treat or activity.

For example, if Mildred is standing at an exit door in the assisted living home anxiously asking, "Where is my son? I'm so worried!," getting her away from the door could be a major problem if you know nothing about her son. When you know the Life Story, you can talk with her about her son, provide reassurance that he is okay, and then redirect or "move her in a different direction" to a safer environment (away from the exit) and to a better place emotionally (joking about her son always being late over a nice glass of milk and cookies).

Working with a New Person

When a person is new to a program (or has a new in-home worker), those early days can be challenging. The person may not be happy about his or her changed situation and may want to go home (or fire the in-home worker). Be sure to know some key Life Story bits of information in these early days. For example, an in-home worker who knows that his new client loves sports will have a lot to work with planning shows to watch on T.V. or talking about favorite teams. Virginia emphasizes this in her work at the Best Friends™ Day Center: "When we can just discover a few special interests, talents, habits, or preferences, we can use those to make the early days warm and welcoming."

However, just offering a snack or treat does not build a relationship! Taking a moment to ask what's wrong, showing concern and affection, and talking with the person will help him or her feel heard and understood. After you've taken these few minutes to be present for the person, then offer a nice treat or beverage. This is the art of redirection done the Best Friends way.

Step Three: Working Together to Address Behavior

Behavior will be addressed more effectively when team members work together:

- Get everyone on the same page.
- Have a Three New Ideas Meeting.

Get Everyone on the Same Page

When a person is new to a program or having a behavioral challenge, we sometimes find that each family or staff member is responding differently. This can work against good dementia care. For example, one staff member may artfully redirect someone who wants to exit from his assisted living community, while another simply says, "You can't go there!" If the care team brainstorms and coordinates its approach, and develops some common language or script, the whole team can respond to the situation more artfully. For example, staff can ask the resident about his work as an artist or mention that his son will be visiting soon and then redirect him to an art-related activity or a tour of the art hanging on the walls.

Virginia's favorite message for someone new to a residential setting or day center is that the family or doctor wants him to be here to "build your strength." This isn't a lie, since so often the person needs more physical activity. It's very life affirming and hopeful for the person to feel that he or she has a job to do (e.g., walk, exercise, take care of himself) while adjusting to a new care setting.

Have a Three New Ideas Meeting

When the team is struggling, try getting a small group together for a Three New Ideas meeting. Encourage the group to brainstorm ideas about a challenging situation and see if the team can agree on three new approaches or ideas. David recalls a meeting regarding a woman who had developed a habit of putting objects and papers into the toilet bowl in her room and then flushing. This was causing flooding and damage to the plumbing. Staff kept trying to monitor her and remind her to use the bathroom, but even the best program can't watch someone 24/7. From a Three New Ideas meeting came the idea to turn off the small water valve beneath the toilet bowl in her room between uses. This way, if she did put shoes and socks in the bowl and flush, it would at least minimize the damage. The staff wagered that she wouldn't have the wherewithal to turn the water valve on and off on her own. This idea helped make a challenging situation better.

When Everything Is Going Wrong

When speaking at conferences, answering e-mails, or blogging, we are often asked how to approach situations that are deeply challenging. Some persons with dementia exhibit dangerous aggressive behavior that threatens their own safety or frightens the people around them. What can you do in these situations?

First, we recommend doubling back on the person's medical history and diagnosis. Do you have complete and accurate information? Families sometimes don't know the whole story or don't tell you everything about a person's past mental health history or substance abuse. Did the person have a good medical evaluation? Does the person have frontotemporal dementia, which can cause deep personality changes? Are frightening hallucinations a result of Lewy body dementia? (See the sidebars on these two diagnoses.) Is the person taking a bad combination of medications or psychotropic medications that aren't working? Sometimes a thorough evaluation of the medical history and situation can provide some good ideas (e.g., trying an antidepressant if the person hasn't been on one).

Second, we recommend consulting the Life Story or asking the family whether the behavior has long existed or is new. Behavior change may not be possible for a person who has always had a quick temper and been critical and demanding, but if a sweet-natured person is now a tiger, double down on your efforts to find a reason why as well as a solution. This is also a time to review whether staff have access to Life Stories, know them, and are using them. You may find that despite your best efforts, this isn't happening. Regroup and reinvest in making sure the team knows the Life Stories well in order to more artfully redirect and overcome challenges with behavior.

Third, although psychotropic medications are never our first line of defense, in some instances they may be necessary. If you do need to go in this direction, seek out the expertise of a talented geriatric psychiatrist or a geriatrician, and be judicious. To use an old nursing phrase, "start low (with the dosage) and go slow," and evaluate the need for medication on a regular basis.

The Best Friends Approach to Frontotemporal Dementia

Frontotemporal dementia (FTD) is the only dementia that affects more men than women, and the peak age group is those ages 55–65. Some experts suggest that FTD is also responsible for half the cases of dementia under the age of 65.

FTD first affects personality and behavior. The person with classic FTD can become very self-centered and narcissistic (you could call it the "me, me, me disease"). Other symptoms include a lack of empathy for others, outlandish remarks and behavior, and rapid decline in language. Often those with FTD eat lots of sugar. The disease tends to progress rapidly compared with other dementias.

There is no medical treatment for FTD, and the classic dementia drugs, such as cholinesterase inhibitors (e.g., Aricept™), may make behavior worse. Antidepressants have been helpful.

We find that the best approach to FTD is to give the person as much choice as possible, keep him or her active and engaged, and develop some common scripts to handle challenges. For example, one man with FTD became sexually suggestive with the female staff in his assisted living community. Each staff member was reacting differently to his advances, some laughing it off with a light touch, some fumbling awkwardly to respond, and some losing their temper and responding with shaming words.

After realizing that varying reactions were only making matters worse, the group agreed to adopt a common response: "Hands off, George. I'm a married woman." Staff members practiced the line ahead of time to become comfortable using it. Once their campaign began, George's behavior gradually began to diminish. A drama-free, calm, and consistent response turned the situation around.

Changes in Lewy Body Dementia

Although Lewy body dementia (LBD), named after Dr. Frederick Lewy, has many similarities to Alzheimer's disease, LBD seems to damage executive functioning (i.e., the ability to plan, analyze, or think abstractly). People with LBD also have movement problems similar to those of Parkinson's disease and are sometimes misdiagnosed with Parkinson's. People with LBD have changing wakefulness; they physically go "in and out" throughout the day. They may also have more changes in short-term memory than a person with Alzheimer's disease, surprising you with good days or good moments.

Profound hallucinations are an early and ongoing symptom and are typically visual but can also include sounds and smells. Hallucinations can be a source of amusement or agitation and fear for those with LBD. David worked with a family in which the husband, Marty, would at times see three little people and talk with them. Fortunately, he seemed more amused than upset, although it was clear that he was confused about the reality of his perception. When Marty asked David whether he, too, could see his three friends, David's diplomatic response was, "I don't see your friends, but I believe that you do." This seemed to satisfy Marty.

Fourth, take an honest look at your training programs. Are you working hard to give your team enough skills in supporting the person with dementia? Sometimes care partners have not had enough training and are making mistakes. An outside consultant or support from a reputable group such as the Alzheimer's Association can provide additional training and feedback for your team.

Intimacy and Sexuality in Dementia

In the Dementia Bill of Rights, we share our view that persons with Alzheimer's disease or other dementia have "the right to have welcomed physical contact, including hugging, caressing, and hand-holding" (see Chapter 1). Intimacy that arises from deep friendships, relationships within family, and closeness with a partner is something almost all of us desire.

Sexual intimacy, however, is one of the hardest parts of life to talk about. In fact, discussing sex in relation to persons with dementia remains such a taboo topic that it's omitted from many dementia care training materials, which represents a real disservice to staff. Intimacy and sexuality deserve to be talked about openly, so that all staff can navigate tricky situations with compassion and common sense instead of discomfort or drama.

Staff members benefit from good training and sensitive care planning when it comes to working with a potentially embarrassing situation, such as encountering a person engaged in masturbation or an act of intimacy with their own spouse or partner, or receiving a sexual approach from a person who has lost some of his inhibitions or confuses you with a past (or present) girlfriend or boyfriend, spouse or partner.

Our recommendation: Take a deep breath and speak honestly, setting aside stigma and embarrassment. Be sure that a staff member isn't panicking if two residents are holding hands or offering a kiss. As Virginia says, "Take away the drama, and let's talk about it." Get out your organization's or community's policies on sexuality and intimacy and start training. If these policies don't exist, encourage your organization to develop progressive, clear, and person-centered guidelines.

When it comes to resident-to-resident interactions, there are more grounds for caution and concern. For example, a person with dementia living in a secure memory care assisted living community generally can't give informed consent to engage in a sexual relationship. Resident-to-resident sexual issues can be considered acts of abuse or even assault in some situations and under some interpretations by regulators or law enforcement. Relationships between residents can be especially problematic if one or both people have a spouse. When former Supreme Court Justice Sandra Day O'Connor's husband was a resident at the Beatitudes Campus in Arizona, he found companionship with another woman. In this case, both families supported the relationship because it made both partners happy. But not every family will respond in the same fashion.

Most long-term care companies feel that a potential or ongoing sexual relationship between two residents should be treated with respect and care but also must be disclosed early on to family members. Here, you should use your collective wisdom. Is the relationship a good situation, or is one partner potentially taking advantage of the other? Can you work with the relationship and support it as a dignity and quality-of-life issue, or is it something that should be discouraged?

A Five-Point Plan for Responding to Sexual Situations

When a person makes a sexual advance toward you or you as a care partner find yourself uncomfortable in responding to a sexual situation, try following these five steps:

1. Take a deep breath, center yourself, and make an effort to respond with calmness and empathy.
2. Think about all of the training and reading you've done about dementia care. Recognize that dementia lessens inhibitions and can also cause mistaken identity. The person, for example, may think you are a significant other. Don't shame the person or label him or her.
3. Talk to your supervisor and team. Assess whether the behavior is something that falls within the person's rights (e.g., being with his or her partner or engaging in sexual self-expression). In those cases, create private space. If the behavior is something that should be discouraged (e.g., disrobing in public), work with your team to find ways to cue and redirect. If the behavior involves potential abuse or physical harm from one resident to another or you have other serious concerns, involve appropriate supervisors, care planning teams, and legal or regulatory resources to gain further insights and identify options.
4. Bring the family or person granted power of attorney into the situation early. Provide them with education and encourage a calm discussion of options.
5. Develop affirming language to redirect the person, such as "Bob, I'm not your wife. I'm Joanne, the med tech helping you with your medicines. Here, take a look at this picture of your wife, Linda. She is quite beautiful! Tell me about Linda. I hear she loved to dance and is the life of the party!"

Protecting Yourself from Aggression

Persons with dementia are not necessarily violent, but when confusion leads to fright or frustration, angry or aggressive behavior can follow. Even the best care partners can be pinched, kicked, or slapped when things go wrong.

How can you decrease agitation and protect yourself?

- Use your knowledge and instinct to look for triggers for the behavior. Is it something you have inadvertently done? What is the person trying to communicate? Perhaps the person doesn't want to get up and take a shower and pushing for the person to take a shower produces an angry response. Rushing a person through a task can also create frustration, agitation, and anger. Consider whether pain, illness, or an infection (e.g., a urinary tract infection) might be causing discomfort that leads to an aggressive outburst.

- Pay attention to early warning signs, such as frowning, pacing, getting red in the face, punching fists, or shaking one's head in disagreement. In our experience, many incidents that result in staff injuries happen when staff have ignored such signs. If the person is too agitated to take a shower, let it go. The shower can wait until later if it is a matter of safety for you.

- Could another care partner get better results? All of us naturally "click" with certain people but with others not at all. Perhaps another care partner can step in. It's not a sign of failure, just differences in how people relate to each other. A person often has favorites among the staff. If a person doesn't get along with a particular staff member, be creative. Make sure Joanie gives the shower if the person doesn't like Theo.

Avoiding Judgmental Language

Labeling or judging behavior never helps. Staff members will sometimes label a resident as "one of the problem ones," "a feeder," or a "hoarder." This sets up a negative atmosphere, focuses on losses instead of strengths, and is blameful and disrespectful. Think about the time in junior high school when you were given an unpleasant or teasing nickname or even in your adult life if you were on the receiving end of a disrespectful label like "woman driver." Was there a time when someone asked you, "Have you gained weight?" Language can be hurtful and, in the case of dementia, reinforce negative stereotypes and stigmas.

We like a resource from Australia that is part of that country's efforts to build dementia-friendly communities. The "Dementia Language Guidelines" suggest that appropriate language should be "accurate, respectful, inclusive, empowering and non-stigmatizing." Instead of calling a behavior "hopeless" or "impossible," try discussing a behavior as "life challenging" or as an expression of unmet need. As we have practiced throughout this book, the guidelines also remind us to talk about the "person" or "persons" with dementia, not persons who have lost their mind. You can access this instructive document at https://fightdementia.org.au/sites/default/files/full-language-guidelines.pdf.

Bringing It All Together: Patricia Estill

Patricia Estill enjoyed being at the Best Friends™ Day Center and thrived there even late into her journey with dementia. When she began to lose her language skills, she would suddenly vocalize noises and words very loudly. This can be a common occurrence in later-stage dementia and can be very disturbing to those around the person. Sure enough, other day center participants were very upset by the sounds Patricia made.

Applying the three-step approach, we first analyzed the situation and realized that the stimulation of the larger group would sometimes trigger Patricia's vocalizations. We assessed her for pain and other health problems to rule them out. It was clear that her behavior was caused by the impact of dementia on her language centers.

Second, looking at her Life Story, we knew she loved music and art activities. We brought this background information to a staff brainstorming session—our third step. Discussing Patricia's situation, we decided to encourage her art skills. We also decided to try keeping her away from the overstimulation of the whole day center group by having her spend more one-on-one time with a staff member or volunteer. The result? Encouraging her to paint and listen to music paid off. When she was absorbed in these activities and not overstimulated by others, she was happy and rarely vocalized. The Best Friends approach helped move Patricia from tough times to better times.

As shown in Figure 2.1 (see Chapter 2), loss, sadness, and even fear are common emotions among people like Patricia and others with dementia. However, when we surrounded Patricia with Best Friends care partners, we could shift her emotions to a more positive place. Loss turned to fulfillment when her art was framed and displayed, sadness turned to cheerfulness with hugs and compliments, and fear turned into security when she could sense she was surrounded by Best Friends.

Conclusion

If you have been practicing the Best Friends approach, using the Life Story with care, learning the Knack, and engaging the person with creative and meaningful activities, you have already created a therapeutic environment where behaviors that are challenging for staff are lessened. You are experiencing success. Personal care is going well. You have also experienced success with turning *no* into *yes*.

But bad days happen to people with dementia. So do bad moods. It's important to recognize that persons with dementia are more vulnerable to tough times because they live in a world where there can be a lot of confusion and stress. With the Best Friends approach, we hope that these moments are few and far between and that for every day that makes you want to go into the break room and scream, there are many more days that will go well.

We strongly believe in savoring your successes. Perhaps it was someone who at first always wanted to go home and eventually settled in beautifully and truly enjoyed living in your community. Perhaps it was someone who refused personal care and who now not only accepts but enjoys it. What turned things around? Write down your success stories so you can pass on what you've learned in staff meetings and when training new staff.

In our years in dementia care, we have found that we can address challenging behaviors with success more than 90% of the time. Unfortunately, sometimes the journey of dementia creates a very troubling and difficult road for an individual. In these cases, keep trying! The Best Friends approach won't necessarily solve all of your challenges, but it will never make matters worse.

PART 3

Creating and Sustaining a Best Friends Program

By now, you have begun to understand why relationship-centered care, embodied in friendship and respect, is so critical to high-quality dementia care. But not everyone does! Change can be difficult, and there are many barriers to success. Fortunately, there are ways to overcome resistance and embrace the Best Friends philosophy in your care setting.

This final section discusses the tools you can use to begin transforming your care setting's culture into one that embraces the Best Friends™ approach. We begin by addressing the concerns and issues of family care partners. Almost all staff members in memory care settings spend significant time relating to families, which can represent some of our best times on the job as well as the most challenging! Best Friends not only develop empathy for and an understanding of family issues, but also practice strategies to address families who are in denial about what their loved one is experiencing or who may put up roadblocks for success.

This section goes on to offer lots of ideas and best practices for kicking off or enhancing a volunteer program. Supplementing well-trained staff with the talents of energetic and motivated volunteers who bring their life experiences and talents to your care setting is an option worthy of consideration for achieving truly excellent memory care.

The closing chapters bring it all together with an extended discussion about how to create and sustain your Best Friends program and by reminding us of how we, too, benefit when we serve as Best Friends.

CHAPTER 8

Being a Best Friend to Family Care Partners

When we visit dementia care programs around the country, we hear a lot about relationships with family members. Staff members tell us about wonderful family care partners who are supportive of staff and are true Best Friends to their family member. But for every family like this, there are always a few who are overly critical and disruptive, who inject their own family feuds into the care setting, and who inadvertently trigger agitation in the person. Some remarks we have heard from staff members include:

> *They don't seem to understand how hard our job is.*
>
> *Even if we do 100 things right, they focus on the one mistake.*
>
> *It kills me that she argues and corrects her mother—she just doesn't get it that her mom has dementia. After the daughter leaves the mother is agitated for hours.*
>
> *I'm actually afraid of that family. I don't like to admit it, but I go the other way when I see them coming!*

To help defuse and overcome this tension, let's explore what's underneath. This chapter invites you to understand the family experience in the journey of dementia and then try out new strategies for relating to difficult family members. In various places, we have highlighted the excellent advice of our colleague and fellow Best Friends Expert Trainer, Tonya Cox, who is currently administrator of The Homeplace at Midway (Midway, Kentucky) and has years of experience educating both professional care staff and families of people with dementia. We hope that whatever your experience, by the end of this chapter you believe as we do that families need a Best Friend, too.

Family Caregiving and Dementia

Open your daily newspaper or social media page, go to a party, or take part in a service at your faith community and you'll meet families providing care for people with Alzheimer's or other dementia. The U.S. Alzheimer's Association and other sources routinely update their eye-popping figures that millions of family members—most of them women—provide billions of hours of unpaid care to loved ones with dementia. The toll on these family members can be profound, with tremendous physical, emotional, and financial strain and stress. Nearly 60% of family care partners report very high stress, and one-third report symptoms of depression.

Keeping this in mind, always assume that the family members you relate to have traveled a difficult path before they came to you for help. They may have experienced:

• *Grief and loss:* It can be devastating to lose the relationship you once enjoyed with a mother, father, husband, wife, partner, friend, or other relative. Most of the dementias are slow moving, so families have had to cope with years of challenges, such as Mom leaving the bath water running and flooding the house, Dad not paying bills, or a sister jeopardizing her health by eating poorly and failing to take medications correctly.

• *Fear:* Because everyone with Alzheimer's disease and other dementias is a bit different, it's hard for family members to know what the future will bring. Will care go on for 3 years or 13? Might the person leave the house late at night and be injured? Will the family be able to manage the challenges of providing personal care? What if something happens to the primary care partner, or the care provider isn't able to handle the person? As one family told us, "My dad is so grumpy that I'm afraid the in-home worker will quit."

• *Isolation:* Care partners often tell us that friends and family "fall away" and social networks unravel when dementia is in the picture, contributing to isolation and loneliness. It can also be hard for couples when one has dementia and the other is the care partner. One woman told us, "It's too hard to bring my husband with me to the functions we've always attended. Maybe it's just me, but it seems like I'm a third wheel now when I attend an event without him. I don't feel comfortable now in situations where I used to thrive."

- *Family conflict:* Brothers and sisters or the extended family are often not on the same page. One brother may be in denial and think Mom can successfully live at home while a sister thinks she would be happier and safer in assisted living. Sometimes the job of caregiving falls on one family member disproportionately. Old antagonisms flare, and resentments and disappointments can grow. As one daughter put it, "I'm doing all the work and my siblings are doing nothing, but somehow I've become the bad guy."

- *Guilt:* The best care partners often feel the most guilt for the times they said the wrong thing or for making tough decisions (taking away the car keys or checkbook), often against the wishes of the person. As guilt continues, it can damage the care partner's sense of well-being and confidence and contribute to depression. Guilt can also block family members from using needed services.

- *Health concerns:* Sometimes a family member who is 70 is caring for a family member who is 90, or a frail older adult is the primary care partner for a spouse. It's one thing to provide care when you are feeling 100% and another when you have your own chronic health problems or a bad back. Family members immersed in care may also neglect their own health—not exercising, not going to their own doctors regularly, or eating poorly. It's no accident that the "healthy spouse," worn down by the demands of care, sometimes dies before the spouse with dementia.

- *Financial stress:* Alzheimer's disease and other dementias can cost a family its life savings. The cost of care is growing, and a family using services can spend tens of thousands of dollars a year. Even when family members provide much of the care directly, they often have had to leave their job or cut back hours, risking their own long-term financial security.

As you look at this list, think about your own experiences. You may have cared for an older relative or friend, perhaps one with dementia, or for a younger person with a chronic health or other condition. You know that being a care partner has its rewards but can also be tough.

Advice on Relating to Families

Families who are going through their own experience of dementia need a Best Friend, says Best Friends Expert Trainer Tonya Cox.

Just like the person with dementia, they are experiencing grief, fear, and anxiety. Some have been living in a state of unresolved grief for 10 to 20 years. That's a significant state of loss that adds a great deal of stress to their situation. Others are in denial. As staff, we need to meet families where they are, and be compassionate, supportive, loving, and caring. We can't be judgmental. It's our job to help them on their journey, even if they don't fully accept that journey.

The elements of Knack can help us journey with family members just as much as with the person with dementia. We can help families with what we know. We can give them tools to be successful when they are floundering. Remembering that the Best Friends approach is relationship centered, we can create relationships with the family. Like any relationship, it will have its ups and downs. Sometimes it will be tough, and we will have to work through that. But more often, when we have created a strong connection with the family, it will be mutually supportive and productive. The relationship with the family is a journey, too!

As Best Friends care partners, we have developed an understanding of and empathy for people with confusion, memory loss, and other cognitive difficulties related to dementia. Developing our understanding and empathy for their families is just as important. Although most families we work with are appreciative, some bring a lot of baggage that is made worse by the stress and strain they have experienced. When possible, respond with understanding and patience. Hopefully the next day will be a better one for them.

Once in a while a truly difficult family member may not respect boundaries or inappropriately take out his or her anger on the staff. In a Best Friends program, your supervisors will not throw you and your team under the bus. They will be there to give that staff member feedback or to discuss boundaries with even the most unruly family member ("Yell at me if you must, but not at my staff").

Supporting Families

There are a number of steps you can take to support family care partners. After all, you do share a common goal: to bring quality of life to the person and to experience success as you navigate the challenges involved in dementia care. You and your organization or company can help families when you:

- encourage education and learning
- start a support group
- respect diversity
- watch your boundaries
- keep your promises
- model the Best Friends™ approach
- are really good at what you do

Encourage Education and Learning

It's a good idea to create a small lending library or resource center in your care setting. Offer educational materials that can be taken home or checked out. The more the family members know about Alzheimer's disease and other dementias, the better. Many programs promote workshops sponsored by a local Alzheimer's association or university. When these opportunities come up, encourage family members to attend.

The benefits of education cannot be overstated. An educated family is more likely to accept the situation and partner with staff to create a dignified and successful life for the person.

Start a Support Group

Support groups can be rich forums for education and social support, especially for families who have been isolated by caregiving. They represent a safe place to share feelings of frustration, guilt, or fear and to encounter "lessons learned" from families who have been providing care for more years. Whenever possible, offer your own support group or affiliate with a local group sponsored by the Alzheimer's Association (or other reputable organization or agency).

David Troxel recalls attending a support group in which a man shared his guilt over having moved his wife into memory care assisted living. The other family members were supportive and gave him very candid feedback. "You did all you could for years. You didn't have another option. This is the best thing for both of you." As the conversation continued, the husband began to process the feedback and share how much this was helping. "I feel that you are saving my life. Thank you for your acceptance and helping me feel good about this tough decision. Without your help, I might have made the ill-advised decision to take her home tonight."

Virginia Bell notes that families can talk directly with each other and give sometimes challenging and very direct feedback. "They can say, 'you are making a big mistake' or 'get your husband to the memory disorder clinic'—things we can't always say to them as professionals. The group problem solving and candid give and take with other families can be very helpful."

Respect Diversity

Families come in all shapes and sizes today. As you work with families, remember that not everyone has been married or had children. Some people may be supported by a grandchild, cousin, or even a caring neighbor or friend. Some have good relationships with family members, and others may be estranged from children or siblings. Don't assume that someone you've just met comes from a happy all-American family as portrayed on a classic television situation comedy.

The families you serve also come from a variety of cultures. To successfully provide service and care, it's important to understand various cultural traditions. For example, dementia continues to carry a lot of stigma in some cultures. Knowing this may help you to adopt a lighter touch when, for example, having a conversation with family about memory loss. You can start the conversation broadly before introducing a particular aspect of a diagnosis. Some cultures may view accepting help from nonfamily members as shameful. These groups might benefit from a discussion about how your program improves quality of life in ways that families may not be able to achieve. The Alzheimer's Association has educational materials in many languages, and individual chapters in larger cities offer culturally competent training and support for serving diverse communities.

Today, many people have a same-sex partner or spouse. These families want to be sure that your organization is welcoming to the lesbian, gay, bisexual, and transgendered (LGBT) community. The journey for families is hard enough without facing discrimination or additional stigma. One resource for training and education is SAGE, the nation's oldest service and advocacy organization for LGBT older adults (www.sageusa.org).

Depending on where you live, you will also meet people with dementia and family members from diverse religious and faith communities. When serving someone from a faith tradition that might be new to you, use it as an opportunity for personal learning and growth. Virginia recalls a participant in the Best Friends™ Day Center, Masako, who was Buddhist. "When we talked to her about her traditions and placed a small bronze Buddha in her hand, it seemed to help her regain her sense of calm and contentment."

Do what you can to be sure that your organization has developed training and services that are respectful of differences. A Best Friends care partner is welcoming to all.

Watch Your Boundaries

Families will sometimes try to get you to weigh in on medical issues or family conflict. A family member might ask, for example, "What have you heard about coconut oil? Could it help?" or "Do you think my sister needs to visit more?" Be careful. Even if you mean well, your recommendation to try the coconut oil could be seen as medical advice (and what if the person has a bad reaction to the coconut or another supplement?). In the second situation, if you innocently agree that the sister could visit more, it might be reported back to the sister as, "The whole staff thinks you are not doing what you need to do."

There is an old saying that people ask for advice for only two reasons: when they've made up their minds and want someone to agree with them or when they want someone to blame when things go wrong. The Best Friends team embraces a principle from the social work field: Give families good information and options and empower them to make their own decisions, but don't tell them what they should do.

Keep Your Promises

We all like it when friends, work colleagues, or companies we do business with keep their promises. Similarly, families appreciate our best efforts to follow through with our commitments. If you promise that you will get the DVD player fixed by the weekend, make it happen!

At the same time, don't promise something you can't deliver or that is beyond your control. If a family complains that housekeeping is not doing a good job, refer the complaint to the housekeeping director or program manager. If a family member asks you about a bill, direct him or her to the business manager.

In most programs there is a chain of command. Let families know the best person to speak with about any given issue.

Model the Best Friends Approach

Families watch what Best Friends staff members do. Among the family members who visit your program, perhaps you have a husband who endlessly argues or corrects his wife, or a daughter-in-law who says, "Mom can't do anything." Instead of telling those people what they are doing wrong, try modeling the better approach. If your in-home client says he's 40, not 80, let the wife hear you reply how you admire his youthful spirit instead of "What? No, you're not!" If the daughter-in-law is visiting your memory care neighborhood, turn around her negative attitude by letting her see you warmly invite Mom to an afternoon exercise or music class.

When a family sees you give their mother a sincere and enthusiastic compliment and then notices her broadly smiling and offering you a hug, you have created a moment of success that ideally the family members will begin to copy.

Be Really Good at What You Do

When families have confidence in you and your team, they will recognize you as an authority and let you guide them in this long journey. Consider the following story from our book *The Best Friends Staff:*

> The husband of a new resident at Villa Alamar in Santa Barbara had purchased a beautiful new bathrobe for his wife when she moved into memory care. A few days later, he discovered that another woman was wearing his wife's bathrobe. He hit the roof, angry that staff had allowed this to happen.
>
> Jackie Marston, Villa Alamar's talented founding Executive Director, explained that the community was a world of Alzheimer's and other dementia. Possessions like robes tended to move around. If it didn't upset his wife, staff would leave things be until they had an opportunity to put things back later in the day. The husband remained unhappy for several weeks as the bathrobe moved around. When he complained, Jackie gave him the same answer.
>
> One day he came in, saw another woman wearing the robe, and suddenly understood. Jackie's confident and consistent words sunk in. He went up to the other resident and said, "What a beautiful robe! Someone with very good taste must have given it to you!" Jackie, who is a confident and experienced dementia expert, helped him travel from denial to acceptance.

A Neuropsychologist Can Help Get Family Members on Board

Families are often in denial about what is happening to Mom or Dad. This usually goes away over time (it's hard to stay in denial if Mom is wandering off at night or her toothbrush turns up in the freezer). But in some cases, denial remains strong. A family member in denial can delay needed planning, continue to let the family member (unsafely) drive, or resist in-home help, day center services, or a needed move from independent senior living to memory care.

One solution is to encourage a neuropsychological evaluation that can provide a written report about the person's cognitive abilities and capacity. To evaluate someone's memory, neuropsychologists use many strategies, from having the person draw a clock to asking him to name items you might find in a kitchen or animals you might see in a zoo. The results can be very helpful for families divided over Dad's condition. If two siblings think Dad has Alzheimer's and three are sure that nothing is wrong, a written report that describes the father's cognitive losses can be a wake-up call that moves the family toward accepting and dealing with Dad's condition.

Encouraging Early Use of Services

One important way to support families is to encourage early use of services for the person with dementia. Families often wait and wait to use services. The day center might be three blocks away, but a family member might still say, "Mom isn't ready."

Be sure to stress the benefits to the person. When families try to do everything themselves, it often leads to the person or care partner becoming isolated. Stress that an in-home worker, day center, or residential care setting can encourage proper personal care, good nutrition, and valuable socialization.

It's also good to share with families that their caregiving role doesn't go away. It changes. Instead of struggling with personal care, they can delegate that to a trained staff member, freeing up time for family members to have more fun times with their loved one and enjoy activities with engagement.

Sharing your success stories in a way that helps overcome fears may also help. "Mr. Smith was reluctant to have his wife join the day program, but when he did, he found that his wife was happier and he was healthier." Or, "Bob was sure his dad wouldn't adjust to the move to memory care, and now he is one of our most successful residents."

Here's how Tonya Cox supports families in this decision:

> When I meet a family, I spend a lot of time talking about where they are and what is happening. What is their understanding of the situation? How much support do they have? When everything is on the table, I encourage them to make a 6-month plan to tackle immediate needs like lining up a driver for errands or correcting glaring safety issues. Later, we can make a 2-year plan or even plan further into the future. This process helps remove an element of anxiety.

We especially like the way Tonya lowers the pressure by dividing the planning and response into smaller pieces that the family can implement over time. That's a Best Friends care partner in action!

Best Friends Approach to Family Interactions

What follows are a few scenarios with family care partners in which we apply some of the key concepts for being a Best Friend. Watch as Best Friends staff use Knack and demonstrate empathy, understanding, and some creative approaches to potentially challenging family interactions.

A Family Member Doesn't Complete the Life Story Materials or Form

Despite the orientation from the sales and marketing director and follow up from the memory care coordinator, Sue has yet to fill out the Life Story forms relating to her mother. Instead of continuing to pursue an approach that has failed or expressing frustration with the daughter, a Best Friends care partner:

- *Practices empathy:* Understanding that the daughter is overwhelmed, staff arrange a phone interview, relieving her of the responsibility of completing the form on her own.
- *Spends time with the person:* Staff spend time with Mom noting as much information as possible. Talking to Mom is also a nice opportunity for engagement.
- *Asks visitors to help:* Perhaps Mom's minister or next-door neighbor can supply insights or fill in some gaps, like the fact that Mom

was always taking in neighborhood strays or delivered homemade fruitcakes at Christmas.

- *Takes action:* Learning from this experience, a care partner may ask the sales and marketing director to create a Top Ten Card (see Figure 3.3) at the start of the intake process so the care team has some helpful information to work with on the first day of providing services or support.

With these tips, you can get the important Life Story forms completed.

A Family Member Continually Complains about Care

No matter what the team is doing at the day center, Jeremy's wife always seems to have a negative word. She complains about the meals, about the activities, about the coffee, about the fact that you aren't open on weekends, and more. Staff try to be understanding, but her negativity is wearing down some of the team members. A Best Friends care partner:

- *Reflects* on the wife's comments to see whether improvements are needed, without getting defensive.
- *Recognizes* that the wife is under stress or may have feelings of guilt about using the center.
- *Keeps a sense of humor* and recognizes that all families are different. Maybe the wife is a professional critic!
- *Gets creative* and e-mails the wife pictures of her husband having a good time and actively participating at the day center.
- *Encourages* the wife to attend an Alzheimer's Association workshop or support group.
- *Asks* the center director to meet with the wife to offer some constructive feedback.

With such encouragement, Jeremy's wife may begin to change her approach.

A Daughter Argues and Corrects

It can be painful for staff to watch a family member who doesn't get it and constantly corrects or argues with the person. David recalls a daughter who was always telling Mom how they had replaced the diamonds in her jewelry with fake stones. This seemed to upset and confuse the mother, who enjoyed showing everyone her fine jewelry. A Best Friends care partner:

- *Encourages* the daughter to read materials from the resource library or attend a workshop to learn why correcting Mom is a losing strategy.
- *Invites* the daughter to this month's support group.
- *Asks* the executive director or community social worker to do some gentle coaching or intervention.
- *Models* an approach with Knack, letting the daughter see staff give the mother compliments on her beautiful jewelry. "Mrs. Jacobs, your diamond ring is so beautiful. It really sparkles!"

With this modeling, the daughter may begin to understand that it isn't necessary to correct her mother, and seeing Mom's pleasure in receiving the compliments, she might start giving some, too.

Two Family Members Are Feuding About Dad's Care

A family calls a home care company for help for Mom and Dad. A team member from the home care agency arrives at the house to meet the couple and their two children. It seems clear that the parents could greatly benefit from in-home support, but the children don't agree. The son is very focused on the expense and the daughter on the parents' needs. In this situation, a Best Friends care partner:

- *Is careful not to take sides* or get in the middle of the debate, respecting boundaries and offering only information and support.
- *Encourages the family* to seek counseling or mediation from a trusted party, such as an attorney or clergy member or professional geriatric care manager.
- *Acknowledges the concerns* of the son regarding finances but stresses the benefits of in-home support for his parents' safety and well-being.
- *Educates the family* about the power of socialization, noting how the in-home worker will encourage engaging the parents in exercise, music, walks in the neighborhood, and other activities.
- *Stresses the competency and training* of the in-home workers to support the one parent with dementia.
- *Understands* that families can be stuck or in denial about care decisions and therefore offers to give them time to consider their options and needs. The representative from the agency makes a point to stay in touch with the family.

Three weeks after the initial visit, the children reach out and services begin.

No Dessert for Mom

A daughter has asked the staff in a residential memory care community not to offer Mom dessert because she doesn't want her to gain weight. There is no medical reason for the request, and the mother is actually quite slim. A Best Friends care partner:

- *Lets the daughter know that staff are listening* and are carefully considering her request.
- *Steps back* and talks with the care team about the situation.
- *Thinks about the person* and recognizes that it would be upsetting to be the only one not offered dessert at the table.
- *Considers quality-of-life issues* and what gives that resident a sense of dignity and choice.

After putting their heads together in a team meeting, staff decide to let the daughter know they will be sensitive to her request by not constantly encouraging consumption of sweets and by serving more modest portions. However, the staff's message to the family is clear: If Mom wants dessert while dining with her friends, she will get dessert!

They inform the daughter, "That's not our program philosophy. This is your mother's home, and she is dining with her friends." We particularly like a phrase such as "not our program philosophy" because it affirms that a program has expertise and values.

A Son Says His Dad Can't Do Anything (Or Doesn't Want To)

Persons with dementia often respond positively to the social environment of a group setting or the engagement efforts of a well-trained and confident Best Friend. In contrast, families have often had years of struggle getting their family member to do basic things and may feel defeated. We often hear them say, "Mom won't do anything for me" or "My sister just sleeps—don't bother her." How can we overcome this attitude? A Best Friends care partner:

- *Doesn't give up,* and does a careful assessment of Dad's physical health and cognitive abilities, looking for ways to build on remaining strengths.

The Value of Conflict

Conflict isn't necessarily bad, according to Tonya Cox, and can lead to honest discussions about what a person needs to have a good quality of life. Keeping the person at the center of the discussion is important. So is being able to explain why you are doing what you are doing and how it benefits the person. Say that a daughter complains that Mom hasn't bathed in 3 days. If you can explain that you didn't bathe Mom this morning because care partners noticed she was having a bad day and were letting her relax, the daughter may understand. As Tonya often reminds her staff, "all of us have the same goal: to care for the loved one with dementia. When family and staff collaborate to achieve that goal, we all win."

- *Educates* the son by sharing some past success stories and explaining how people with dementia will sometimes do things for others that they don't do for family members.
- *Models new approaches* for the family by, in this case, encouraging the son to sit back and observe a staff member's interactions with his dad.

With education and encouragement, the son may begin trying again to encourage his father to do things, such as attending a special event or program.

Conclusion

In the Preface to this book, Rita West Paustian recalled how her father used the Best Friends approach to "know just how to engage my mother so that she continued to feel needed and loved."

One of the best ways to be a Best Friend to a family care partner is to help the person find success. When care partners like Rita's father learn all they can about dementia care and practice the Knack—the art of doing difficult things with ease—care almost always becomes easier and more fulfilling.

Feeling effective as a care partner contributes to wellness, confidence, and optimism. It lifts families above some of the stress and negativity that often drags them down. Helping family members experience success helps them feel like they can learn from this tough experience and envision a future in which they can feel a sense of accomplishment and pride about the time they have spent in relationship with the person during the course of the disease.

We know that some family members are really stuck and can't see any hope or feelings of success. These are families who would especially benefit from the Best Friends approach. Seeing staff members model excellent care, experience success, and receive smiles and hugs instead of frowns and slaps can truly transform a family's worldview.

As one daughter recently told us, "I'm so in the moment with Mom. We laugh all the time. Some of our issues from the past have now been forgotten—by both of us. I'm closer to my mom now than I have been in years."

The Best Friends approach helps staff and families come together in common purpose: to bring out the best in the person with dementia while experiencing the benefits of engaging activities, meaningful communication, and shared Life Stories. There will be plenty of challenges along the way but also opportunities for laughter, connection, and love.

CHAPTER 9

Growing a Volunteer Program

Having well-trained staff providing dementia care is critical, but staff can't always be everywhere at once. A Best Friends staff will demonstrate confidence and skills and help create a positive culture, but most programs still face limited resources. One way to improve the care and engagement of persons with dementia in your community is to recruit and train volunteers. Energetic and motivated volunteers bring their life experiences and talents to a dementia care setting. They may play the piano, create and lead art and music programs, accompany groups on field trips, or serve on boards and committees. When you introduce volunteers to the Best Friends™ approach, they do all of the above with the Knack of great care: learning and using Life Stories, managing challenges, and enjoying conversation and connection. Just as the Best Friends philosophy supports quality of life for the person with dementia, it also helps volunteers enjoy successful, meaningful interactions every time they enter your care setting.

We have a special love of volunteers because we have witnessed the richness they add to a program. In the early days of the Best Friends™ Day Center program, Virginia Bell's budget for staff was small. Seeking a creative alternative, Virginia matched volunteers and persons with dementia by interest—farmers with farmers, knitters with knitters, and so on—a significant innovation at the time. These volunteers built deep, rewarding, long-lasting relationships and helped the center come close to providing one-to-one companionship. Drawing from the Life Story, they started conversations on everything from life on the farm to Swedish movies, enlivened ice cream socials and gardening projects, and brought a spark to the program committee that planned themes and activities. Over time, we discovered that the spirits of the persons with dementia and the volunteers were fed by their time together, because the volunteers were seeking relationships, too.

> T.J. Todd, an early Best Friends™ Day Center volunteer, was heartbroken when his friend Dicy died. "You know, we spent so many hours together, hundreds of hours. In many ways I spent more time with Dicy than my other friends outside the program, and when she died I felt such a sense of loss. I really did lose my best friend."

Best of all, working with volunteers helped spread the Best Friends philosophy out into the world. Thousands of students who have volunteered at the center during our 30-year history have become strong advocates for our relationship-based approach. Virginia observes that the program has always served as a "Center of Excellence" and takes great satisfaction from knowing the program has introduced future nurses, social workers, doctors, and others to best practices for dementia care.

> An undergraduate at the University of Kentucky when he first came to the Best Friends™ Day Center, Dr. Peter Reed went on to work for the Alzheimer's Association and serve as executive director of the Pioneer Network, which seeks to change the culture around caring for older adults. Today, he is director of the Sanford Center for Aging at the University of Nevada at Reno. "My time at the day center helped me realize that I wanted to commit my professional life to working with elders," he says. "I learned back then that one key to a successful program is that Virginia and David created a caring environment for all present. Staff, volunteers, families, and, of course, the participants felt loved and valued. It's what culture change is all about and what we strive for in all of our long-term care settings."

Virginia jokes, "We'd like to take some credit for his success!"

Many programs would like to recruit and involve volunteers but don't know where to start or how a volunteer program would work. Developing an effective volunteer program takes focus and planning. The barriers to success can seem overwhelming. Staff leaders are often concerned that volunteers won't be reliable, won't want to go through fingerprinting and tuberculosis tests required by some states, or will simply find the work too difficult. Direct care staff can also be ambivalent, feeling that they are already too busy and that volunteers might add more burden to their already challenging work life. One executive director of an assisted living community summed it up for us when she said, "Volunteers—that's on my to-do list."

This chapter offers program leaders insight into volunteerism as it relates to dementia care and shares Virginia's best practices for success in encouraging volunteers to join your Best Friends community. If you are not in a decision-making role, you'll still find good ideas on how to relate to and nurture volunteers in your care setting. Many of the ideas in this chapter came from an interview with Virginia Bell conducted by David Troxel for Eldercare Conversations (see the Suggested Resources under "Activity Resources and Programming").

Effective Volunteerism

The United States has a rich history of volunteerism. In 1736, Benjamin Franklin founded the first volunteer firehouse. In the 1800s, many religious groups began charitable efforts, and groups such as the YMCA/ YWCA and Red Cross were founded. In the 1900s, service clubs such as the Rotary Club and Lions Club began. More recently, the nonprofit Points of Light Foundation and the Corporation for National and Community Service (CNCS), an independent federal agency, promote and support volunteerism. As a result of this legacy, the United States has a unique interest and success record when it comes to volunteerism. According to CNCS, every year Americans give nearly 8 billion hours of volunteer time. One in four adults volunteers through an organization doing fundraising, building or repairing houses, serving meals at homeless shelters, singing in church choirs, and tutoring or teaching.

In dementia care or service settings, volunteers serve on nonprofit boards and committees, raise money at special events and walks, take part in speakers bureaus, do office work, and facilitate support groups. They also engage in relationships with people with dementia, participating alongside them in activities, providing hands-on support and care, and even providing respite care. Informal volunteers may support a friend or family member with dementia outside of a formal organization.

As the late American humorist Erma Bombeck once said, "Volunteers are the only human beings on the face of the Earth who reflect this nation's compassion, unselfish caring, patience, and just plain loving one another." Yet in order to be compassionate and caring, volunteers need structure. Those Habitat for Humanity houses? Before anyone shows up with a hammer, hundreds of hours have been invested in organizing the project so that all participants have clear roles that match their interests and skills. Without that effort, volunteers might just mill around on the edges, wondering why they are there or what they should do first.

To flourish, volunteers also need support from capable staff. Volunteers aren't free labor! They are not a way to compensate for poor staffing or poor programming. When the basics are in place, what volunteers offer is enrichment that helps take your program to new levels of excellence.

Let's take a look at some of the tasks involved in preparing your program for the presence of volunteers.

Steps to Starting a Successful Volunteer Program

There are a number of steps you can take to build a successful volunteer or student program:

- Write a purpose statement for your volunteer program.
- Do a self-assessment and set goals for your program.
- Develop job descriptions.
- Creatively recruit and interview.
- Provide meaningful orientation and training.
- Create a satisfying experience.
- Say thank you in many ways.

Write a Purpose Statement for Your Volunteer Program

If you are just starting out, get a small group together and spend a few hours brainstorming and talking about your vision for a volunteer program. Use your results to create a short purpose statement or description of your proposed (or revised) volunteer program.

As you write this program description, consider how a Best Friends philosophy can be used. For example, can you encourage your new volunteer piano player to learn Life Stories in order to play favorite songs? Can you match volunteers and persons with dementia who have similar interests or backgrounds to facilitate time for conversation and connection? What overall benefit will volunteers bring to the program?

Do a Self-Assessment and Set Goals for Your Program

Whether you are developing or expanding your volunteer effort, step back and ask, "Are we ready?" Volunteers add tremendous value and richness to any program, but they take time. Do you have a designated volunteer coordinator or staff person who will take charge of the program? Are you set up to create work assignments, supervise, and evaluate your new volunteers? Have you considered how to introduce them to your Best Friends philosophy, including preparing and using the Life Story and the value of doing things with the person that have meaning and support quality of life?

Another important consideration is staff attitudes. We have seen situations in which staff didn't really want volunteers or didn't understand the role they would be playing. It is necessary to educate staff about why you are recruiting volunteers, reassure them by clarifying roles, and get everyone excited about participating.

Set goals for your program. It's okay to start small. If you are part of a smaller memory care neighborhood in assisted living, consider trying to recruit and train five new volunteers. After these five volunteers are on board, evaluate how things are going. If it's going well, you may be ready to add five more. You can scale up as you learn from your experiences and as your resources permit.

Develop Job Descriptions

It's always important to create a job description, even for the simplest volunteer assignment. Make sure the volunteer fully understands the responsibilities he or she will be assigned as well as how the position is helping your organization and persons with dementia—be it engaging with them (encouraging quality of life) or folding and mailing newsletters (educating the public).

Jobs and roles can be varied. Some are hands-on, such as visiting with residents or assisting with activities. Others support in different ways, such as fundraising or serving on a committee. Volunteers can also help design and support good programming. Field trips and outings, for example, take staff planning and perhaps a "scouting trip" can be used to check for accessible pathways or family-friendly bathrooms. Why not design a role for a volunteer or volunteers who can help create your yearly calendar of field trips or plan monthly art classes or weekly trivia themes? Specific job descriptions will make it easier to recruit volunteers with special talents, such as musicians or retired artists.

As you develop job descriptions, remember that volunteers should never be used to replace paid staff. It's the responsibility of program managers to provide adequate care. Volunteers will jump ship if they feel that they are being exploited or that they are undermining staff in any way.

Simple, Relationship-Based Volunteer Activities

- Read to a person with limited vision.
- Take a walk or push the person in a wheelchair to enjoy a beautiful garden.
- Play board games or enjoy puzzles.
- Work on an art project together.
- Provide respite for a family member caring for a person at home (or visit someone living alone).
- Give a manicure.
- Sing or make music together.
- Spend time talking and reminiscing or "chit-chatting" like old friends.

Creatively Recruit and Interview

Once you have a plan, organizational buy-in, and job descriptions, you can begin to recruit volunteers. We recommend taking several approaches. First is the individual ask. Consider people you know who would make great volunteers (e.g., a friend or family member who plays guitar). Approach the person, talk about your program, and invite him or her to become involved ("Mike, you are so outgoing—would you consider playing guitar for our day center? It would bring so much joy to our participants.").

Virginia has also enjoyed great success asking family care partners to volunteer once they are no longer providing care to their own family member. "Some family members want to take all that they have learned as care partners and help others, even after their family member has died," she says. Look for families who have been highly involved in your program. Families who had energy, kept a sense of humor, brought in goodies for everyone—they can be reluctant to walk away from a program or community that they've enjoyed being a part of.

> Jean Georges of Las Vegas, Nevada, was a care partner to her husband, Leonard, for many years during his journey with Alzheimer's disease. She now volunteers at the Cleveland Clinic Lou Ruvo Center for Brain Health, greeting new patients and families and helping out with the center's educational programs. When David met Jean at the center in Las Vegas, he was struck by her positive energy, smiles, and giving spirit. "She even gave me a ride back to the airport after my talk."

Mining a Life Story can also provide a lot of potential recruits. For example, a resident in assisted living or skilled nursing might have belonged to a sorority, service club, or large faith community, or taught at a local high school. With family consent, visit that local college sorority and invite them to "adopt" that resident, do an educational program at that faith community, approach the high school about their student programs, get on the weekly lunch schedule of that service club. This is how you begin to find success.

One of the easiest ways to recruit is to make a list of special talents that would benefit people in your program. Can you identify a volunteer piano player, artist, or person with a friendly pet therapy dog to begin visiting? Asking this talented person to help your program once a week or several times a month is easy. He or she might enjoy the good feeling that comes from the experience and the many smiles his or her talent will evoke.

In a senior living setting, ask the residents in independent living to "adopt" a Best Friend in the memory care program and visit once a week or on a regular basis. Let prospective volunteers know that regular visits are meaningful and appreciated, even if they are short. A 30-minute visit 50 weeks a year adds up to 25 hours of engagement!

Once a potential volunteer has been identified, conduct a formal interview, much as you would for a prospective employee. The interview should be friendly and encouraging, and it's important to help the potential volunteer understand your program so that both of you can determine whether the person is a good fit. Some states and regulatory agencies require fingerprinting, background checks, and a test for tuberculosis for volunteers. Although it may seem a potential barrier, we find that most volunteers are willing to jump through these hoops.

Virginia notes that some Best Friends™ Day Center staff were fearful that an interview and certain state requirements might dissuade people from volunteering. "In fact, I think it has impressed potential volunteers with our professionalism and makes it even more special when we agree that the volunteer will bring great skills, talents, and heart to our program," she says.

Provide Meaningful Orientation and Training

Volunteers benefit from a robust orientation and ongoing training. This takes commitment, but good training supports confidence and success. Besides covering the basics of dementia and the principles of the Best

Friends Approach, consider topics such as confidentiality, communication, and volunteer dos and don'ts, such as being aware of special diets, not trying to lift someone on your own, and knowing when to call for help.

Quarterly volunteer meetings are an opportunity for additional training and team building. Volunteers can share their stories and meet one another over a nice lunch or snacks while hearing a lecture or workshop about a valuable topic. Guest speakers are a great resource and will often donate their time to speak to a group of community volunteers. Consider inviting local physicians and nurses, staff from a memory disorder clinic or university research center, or a representative of your local Alzheimer's association or society.

Adapt training to specific roles and responsibilities. For example, the new piano player will appreciate understanding the importance of introducing him- or herself, describing the music being played, and playing popular refrains more than once. Repeating key lyrics like "She'll be comin' round the mountain when she comes" during a sing-along will help participants enjoy this memorable phrase and perhaps spark lyrical memories.

Be sure your training draws deeply on your Best Friends philosophy. Let volunteers know that your program values relationships and connection and that all of you are working to create a therapeutic environment that is life affirming and fun.

Create a Satisfying Experience

For more than 30 years, the Best Friends™ Day Center has drawn volunteers who spend a morning or afternoon once a week with an assigned Best Friend. More than 100 volunteers are active in the program at any given time, defying conventional wisdom that volunteers won't make this kind of commitment. Why does the program succeed? Virginia believes it's because the center offers volunteers "a satisfying experience."

Making sure the work is significant is the best way to ensure a satisfying experience. At the Best Friends™ Day Center program, volunteers work one-on-one with people with dementia, generally one (4-hour) morning or afternoon a week. As they spend time together walking, talking, or enjoying a snack or meal, volunteers can see the impact they have on their Best Friend. Volunteers can easily understand the significance of their role and how it affects the center as well as the participants with dementia.

Creating and nurturing a group identity is another ingredient of a satisfying experience. Volunteering puts people in a new setting where they can meet others and make new friends. At the Best Friends™ Day Center, volunteers are recruited and trained in "classes." Inviting five or six volunteers to attend an orientation together helps them get to know one another and begin to build bonds that can last a long time.

The Best Friends program also reinforces a sense of group identity by offering regular social functions for the volunteers for each day the center is open. Volunteers in the "Monday group" or "Thursday group" enjoy getting to spend time with one another. To support and educate volunteers, the day program hosts ongoing training and monthly luncheons where volunteers and staff can discuss challenges and share program updates. A volunteer newsletter welcomes new volunteers and celebrates volunteer birthdays and special events.

Virginia notes that this "satisfying" and indeed rewarding experience has led to volunteers working in the program for years. "The day program is now over 30 years old and we still have one volunteer who was there from the beginning. Many of our volunteers have worked 10 years or more. We've become quite a family," she says.

Say Thank You in Many Ways

Although we don't necessarily object to giving gifts to volunteers, the truth is most of us have more than enough mugs, pens, and t-shirts. The best way to thank volunteers is a simple "Thank you."

Organize regular appreciation events, including an annual lunch or dinner. Keep track of hours worked and give certificates acknowledging certain milestones, such as 100 hours or 1 year of service. If your community has a "Local Hero" award or special volunteer issue in the newspaper, take the time to nominate a special volunteer. A volunteer who is honored will feel a sense of pride and accomplishment, and the publicity not only will benefit your program but may also attract other volunteers.

Getting to Five Stars

For a little extra motivation as you grow your volunteer program, imagine how it might be evaluated by online review services such as Yelp or Trip Advisor. What will your new volunteers be saying to their friends after their time with you? Will they be giving your setting high marks?

Authentic Relationship, Satisfying Experience

Tom Meyer has volunteered at the Best Friends™ Day Center for many years. The relationships he has enjoyed with men like Russell Doudt and Bob Steele are the reason he stays involved. Here is how Tom describes his experience:

> Russ Doudt was a waist gunner on a B-17 bomber flying in the Pacific during World War II. We often talked about his experiences, like dealing with junior officers, losing an engine, and the day he was injured in a crash. We laughed about how they obtained booze from the officers' mess and about how important the GI Bill was that allowed him to attend college after the war. One day when shopping for toys with my grandson, I saw models of B-17 and B-25 bombers. I bought these, and Russ and I put them together during several Best Friends sessions. Our plan was to display them in the room where Best Friends meet, but when I did not see them I was told that Russ had taken them home. I have been told they are on a dresser in Russ's bedroom to this day.
>
> Bob Steele and I shared many meaningful memories about being a cadet at the U.S. Naval Academy. We placed small wagers on athletic contests between West Point and Annapolis, we shared memories about places we had both lived during our military careers, and I often reminded him that his father was a colonel in the Army. We shared a common interest in the Civil War and together attended several meetings of the local Civil War Round Table. We continue to share memories, and based on our common background we have the ability to talk about current events and books we have read, and in general enjoy each other's company.

Volunteers such as Tom bring their own special point of view to the Best Friends™ Day Center, where their key "men skills" have appealed to men who would rather occasionally skip an arts-and-crafts session to talk about sports, careers, or military service with another guy.

Involving Student Volunteers and Interns

As schools have instituted community service requirements, many middle school, high school, and college students are seeking volunteer opportunities of an hour or two a week. These opportunities are win-win for everybody. Students can provide a lot of youthful enthusiasm and energy, older adults light up around young people who remind them of their children and grandchildren, and you will be doing your part to educate future professionals about dementia care.

Older students in professional programs may need internships that help them earn significant clinical or practical hours during a semester. You may be approached by:

- social work students who want to attend a family support group to better understand the impact of dementia on family care partners
- medical or nursing students, or certified nursing assistant students, who want to shadow your staff
- students in social work, occupational therapy, speech therapy, or other professional programs who hope to work one-on-one with someone with dementia
- gerontology students who want to participate in a continuing care community
- recreational therapy students who want to create a customized exercise program
- nursing students who want to participate in a program at a day center

Taking part in student or professional training programs takes some coordination and effort. Typically, your organization will need to identify local schools with volunteer or internship programs, meet with the key decision makers, and then work with a volunteer or internship coordinator to design the student experience. Build in an orientation for your new student volunteers and interns that can also cover some basic dos and don'ts.

There may be some program requirements (e.g., writing up an evaluation of the student's work or taking part in a faculty–student meeting). In some cases (e.g., medical students), the volunteer experience may simply involve visiting your program or care setting once and spending time with a person with dementia. In other situations, students may contribute significant hours over a semester or year. The good news is that once you have done the preliminary paperwork and built successful relationships with a school program, you will enjoy years of student contact.

Although many student programs focus on time that students spend with the person with dementia, don't forget that students may also find it helpful to talk with staff and family care partners or even attend a support group meeting.

Your students will enjoy learning about and practicing the Best Friends approach. Celeste Lynch, director of wellness at Moorings Park in Naples, Florida, has noted a significant upswing in student interest since her organization adopted a Best Friends approach. "We are top of their list. The students are intrigued about how Best Friends creates a joyful and successful environment for our residents."

Working with students delivers immediate benefits, and in the long term your key staff and organization can take pride in introducing a new generation of young people to dementia care. Who knows? Maybe one of your young volunteers, like Peter Reed, will be inspired to embrace a career in dementia care and advocacy.

Conclusion

Volunteers bring energy and new points of view to memory care settings. In a well-run volunteer program, volunteers can lift the spirit of paid staff and the people with dementia. They might bring tomatoes from the garden, freshly baked cookies, and lots of compliments and support. They can become an integral part of your Best Friends community.

Starting a volunteer program takes lots of up-front work. At the outset, it might seem like the return on investment (your time) isn't paying off (not enough success), but once you see volunteers becoming dedicated ambassadors for your program, giving loving support to people with dementia, becoming friends with staff, families, and each other, and turning up with those cookies, you will feel that the time invested has paid some great dividends.

CHAPTER 10

Creating and Sustaining Your Best Friends Program

When Moorings Park, a continuing care retirement community in Naples, Florida, implemented the Best Friends™ approach for its residents with dementia, the impact was profound. According to Celeste Lynch, director of wellness: "We've seen great results in our activity programming, staff training, and campus-wide awareness of dementia care. Notably, residents with dementia who weren't participating in activities are now more fully engaged, and staff report that behaviors have declined and cooperation and happiness have increased."

Creating a Best Friends culture at Moorings Park took a focused effort. Celeste Lynch chaired the effort. Step 1 was to send several staff members for training at a Best Friends™ Approach Institute for Master Trainer Certification, which equipped them to become Master Trainers. Next, the newly minted Master Trainers and other staff formed a Best Friends committee that worked across the various levels of care to create a game plan for the organization. Regular meetings and monthly themes kept the team focused on the project and supported shared accountability. The results have been very positive, and a Best Friends culture has gradually taken hold. "Best Friends is helping us establish ourselves as a center of excellence in dementia care throughout our region," says Dan Lavender, Moorings Park president and CEO.

Moorings Park is just one of many long-term care programs around the world that has transformed itself into a community with a Best Friends care culture. These efforts are impressive because change can be difficult,

The Best Friends Environment

In a Best Friends environment, staff:

- contribute to a positive and uplifting atmosphere with smiles and affection
- know and use Life Stories
- always put the person before the task
- develop caring, respectful relationships
- take part in activities with engagement
- accomplish personal care with confidence
- address behaviors that are challenging with creativity
- work as a team, helping each other whenever needed
- know how to use the Knack in their interactions with people with dementia

and there can be many barriers to success. Co-workers can be apathetic, a boss unsupportive, and almost all of us run up against limited time and tight budgets. But it's possible! Along with our own ideas, in this chapter you will hear from professionals from a variety of care settings who have successfully adopted and put into practice Best Friends principles.

What if, in your workplace, you're not the one with the power to implement a change? What if you suspect you may have to go it alone? We'd like to reassure you that we have watched many committed people make a significant impact on their workplace. So even if you are in what Virginia Bell and David Troxel have sometimes called "The Old Idea Program" (described later in this chapter in the sidebar "Old Idea vs. New Idea Programs"), you can become a Best Friends champion.

Steps for Creating a Best Friends Culture

Changing a culture takes time, commitment, and focused effort. Fortunately, it's possible to break the sometimes intimidating process of culture change into smaller, achievable steps. In our experience, the following are the steps needed to start and sustain your program:

- Assess your current program's strengths and areas you want to improve.
- Create a short game plan with measurable goals.

- Organize a Best Friends task force or committee to help you roll out a new approach.
- Develop a 12-month calendar that focuses on one key area each month or quarter.
- Build the language of Best Friends into your program.
- Take staff training to a higher level.
- Sell the benefits.
- Address barriers and objections.
- Celebrate your successes.

Assess Your Current Program

Before you begin, take some time to look at your program, piece by piece. How are things going? What is working? What is not? Convene a small group of staff from several departments (or a diverse group of staff and volunteers) to brainstorm and speak candidly. Use a flip chart on an easel or white board to capture your notes. Here are some of the topics to discuss:

- Is every day a struggle, or are staff having success in managing routine behavior challenges? Target specific challenges, such as unsafe exit seeking or too many falls.
- Are the activities lively, robust, and creative?
- Are staff satisfied? How is turnover? Do you have staff members who are working in the wrong job or who are too negative or overly task oriented? Identify staff who already exhibit Best Friends qualities and instinctively get the Best Friends approach. They will be key allies in your change process.
- What kind of family feedback do you get? Are families happy or disgruntled? If you already conduct an annual family satisfaction survey, read through it closely. If you don't, consider conducting a one-time survey before your meeting.
- What is your census? Full, with a waiting list, or lots of vacancies? This can be a measure of your success (or lack thereof) in the marketplace.
- Does your program measure use of psychotropic medications? How many people are taking them? Can the percentage be reduced?
- If you are an in-home provider, is your staff reporting successes or struggles? Do families call and say they want more hours (a sign that you are meeting their needs)?

- Are you keeping up with important paperwork and care planning?
- Is your program or community meeting its financial goals?

Candidly examining the current program will help you begin to identify concerns, set goals for the future, and create a starting point to measure your future success. For example, the discussion may reveal a need to measure family satisfaction and turnover or to develop a much more robust activity program.

A special note for those who may be going it alone: It's okay to start this work on the back of an envelope or note pad. Don't get overwhelmed. Write down your own perceptions to get started.

Create a Game Plan with Measurable Goals

After noting the main strengths and challenges of your current program, do some thinking about key areas for focused change. Let's say your assessment comes up with the following:

- Life Story forms are incomplete or not prepared at all.
- Several staff report being slapped by residents.
- Activities are going well Monday through Friday, but nights and weekends seem to fall apart.
- Orientation for new employees is uninspired and outdated.
- Strengths: good staff, but they are somewhat task oriented.

Share the list with a small group or with the leadership team and begin to set goals that can be measured. Perhaps you want to focus on activities and engagement for the next 3 months or revamp the process of gathering information for the Life Story. Set down your goals in a one- or two-page game plan and use these to help shape a vision and to-do list.

For example, goals for the five-point list above could include:

1. Create an awareness campaign around Life Stories and dedicate a specific month to writing or refreshing all Life Stories of residents and participants.
2. Develop a 1-hour in-service on resident agitation and staff safety and provide to all staff within 3 months.
3. Increase weekend activity programs by 4 hours a day. Juggle staffing budget to add a dedicated activity person every Saturday and Sunday by the start of the next fiscal year.

4. Work with the human resources department to create a new 4-hour orientation involving lectures and hands-on experience for rolling out a mentorship program.
5. Plan a series of stand-up topics and short trainings on the difference between task focus and person focus.

Creating these goals supports your ability to evaluate your success. For example, if you update the Life Stories of 32 participants during February, and present two stand-ups on how to use them daily, you can consider goal #1 in the list above for Life Stories accomplished. While you're not a research institution, it's important to have some tools to evaluate how your project is going.

Organize a Best Friends Task Force or Committee and Choose a Point Person

Changing a culture is a team effort. Start by creating a Best Friends task force or committee, a group of people within the organization who have the wisdom, experience, and authority to help build and roll out a new program. Encourage diversity on the committee. For example, a nonprofit continuing care retirement community may want to include the chief operating officer, director of nursing or wellness, activities director, marketing director, a CNA or staffer from the program, plus a family volunteer and board member.

The committee should be charged with reviewing and refining the initial goals you've created and coming up with a specific calendar and lists of tasks and activities. Be sure that the committee members are fully on board with the changes ahead. They will be your community ambassadors, providing education and hopefully excitement about the new Best Friends work. Social worker, writer, and educator Dan Kuhn says that a "team of champions" can sell culture change programs and their benefits to all employees of an organization and, once it's under way, help keep the message (and program) alive.

Write a purpose statement for the committee and include it in all of your materials in order to build awareness about the new initiative and to begin building support for the group. Here is a sample purpose statement:

> This work group will develop an action plan to implement key areas of the Best Friends philosophy to improve the quality of life and quality of care for people with dementia. The group will assess our current dementia program, including key elements such as environment, staff training, healthcare, assessment, and

communications and marketing materials. The group will create a timeline and program goals and objectives and will evaluate the results on a regular basis.

Prestige Care in Vancouver, Washington, launched the development of
its new dementia program, Expressions, with a 2-day dementia care
boot camp. The meeting assembled a diverse team of enthusiastic people representing a variety of positions—including CNAs, activity staff,
nurses, administrators, and sales and marketing personnel—to review
and renew its existing memory care program. "The group process
supported buy-in, fostered creativity, and allowed us to hit some key
elements like Life Story out of the ballpark," says Hollie Fowler, senior
director of product and brand development of Prestige Care. Although
the Expressions program is proprietary to Prestige, the Best Friends philosophy has been influential in its development. Expressions has gar-
nered great reviews and awards from the field and helped the company
achieve record census.

Tonya Cox of Christian Care Communities has some encouraging
words for those who aren't experienced in managing change: "It's okay
to be a bit messy and let it evolve. If you get a talented group of people
together with a shared purpose, you'll be surprised how far you can go."
Tonya also encourages designating a Best Friends point person who can
chair your work group, provide resources and support, and be the project
spokesperson. "Particularly in larger care settings or in situations where
a company is doing this work with multiple locations," Tonya notes, "it's
essential for everyone to know who is leading the effort." This person (or
persons, if you have co-chairs) can organize meetings and trainings, keep
the minutes and notes, and provide ongoing leadership for the effort.

Develop a 12-Month Calendar that
Focuses on One Key Area Each Month or Quarter

Even with the best intentions, making progress can be difficult. With
e-mails and other day-to-day responsibilities demanding our attention, it's much easier to react to the crisis of the day than proactively
plan future goals. We recommend breaking the adoption process into
a 12-month calendar of monthly or quarterly activities that the Best
Friends work group or champion can more easily accomplish. The plan
could follow the outline of this book, for example, by focusing on Life
Story review for a month, then on communication the next month. Or
it could support the specific goals you have identified and agreed upon.

It's optimal to have a 1-year plan with a variety of activities to serve as a roadmap for success, but it's also okay to create a more short-term plan. Another idea is to focus on one major area each quarter, with tasks and accomplishments tied to your goals. No matter how long your calendar, be sure to build in time at the beginning to get organized and review internal materials. The following sample 12-month work plan shows how to build in time:

- *Months 1 to 3: Get started.* During this internal planning period, focus on organizing the committee and refining your goals. Make a plan to secure buy-in for the effort from stakeholders, including families and key program leaders.

- *Month 4: Teach the basics of Alzheimer's disease and other dementias.* The first step to rolling out change is to get all staff on the same page around dementia. Use key handouts such as the Dementia Bill of Rights, show short videos, and invite guest speakers.

- *Month 5: Address infrastructure.* Review the physical and care environment for needed changes or improvements. Do you need to budget for new furniture and lighting? Program supplies? Consider revising job descriptions and program forms to reflect the new goals and principles you are pursuing. A residential care program may also need to include content on housekeeping and dining.

- *Month 6: Delve into preparing the Life Stories.* Provide staff education on Life Stories and their importance. Roll out new or revised Life Story forms. (Use the template in Chapter 3.) Write Life Stories on each person. Devise creative ways to share resident Life Stories among all staff.

- *Month 7: Focus on communication.* Practice new ways of communicating by using role-plays. Share Best Friends handouts on good dementia communication strategies. Ask committee members to model excellent communication, such as giving compliments, slowing down while talking, and offering smiles and welcomed hugs.

- *Month 8: Explore behaviors.* Offer renewed training on how to address challenging behaviors. Discuss behavior as a form of communication. Drawing on staff experiences, develop case studies that show how using the Life Story and creative problem solving help reduce behaviors that are challenging. Establish processes for collective problem solving around behaviors (e.g., in team huddles, care planning meetings).

- *Month 9: Include families.* Use this month to offer educational programs on dementia to your families. This is also a good time to train staff about family dynamics and the difficult physical, emotional, and financial challenges that come with being a family care partner.

- *Month 10: Get the Knack.* Use the "Knack–No-Knack" vignettes in Chapter 5 to introduce and practice the concept. Use the Calgary KNACK acronym in Chapter 5 as a motivating poster. Ask staff to share their own Knack and No-Knack stories. Make it fun!

- *Month 11: Develop activities with engagement.* Keep this month informative and hands-on. Train your team on 30-second activities and the importance of meaningful engagement. Invite staff to contribute their best ideas on how your program can add value and richness to the daily life of each person you serve. Consider developing a roster of residents, challenging staff to come up with one person-to-person activity to do the following week. Match your receptionist who loves flower arrangements with a retired florist in your memory care program. Put two football fans together.

- *Month 12: Wrap it up.* Use this month to review all of the preceding work and write a short report restating your goals and listing your achievements. For example, note the successful reworking of Life Stories and how they have paid off in daily care. Highlight new training modules that have been developed. Share positive reactions from the staff and family members.

With this, or some other, 12-month plan in hand and your strategies lined up, you will be ready to jump in! Some months and topics will go better than others, but having a clear and simple plan like the one above makes implementation easier and helps keep everyone focused on the goals that have been set. Be sure to roll out this monthly campaign with some flourish. Create some posters, prizes for staff, monthly activity supplies, and other items to draw attention to the ongoing campaign and to keep everyone's focus on the effort.

Build the Language of Best Friends into Your Program

Help implement a Best Friends program by using the Best Friends vocabulary throughout your campaign so it becomes an everyday practice. By this we mean use the key terms and foundational concepts presented in the Introduction. Here are some examples of ways to adopt Best Friends vocabulary:

"I'm Mike. I'm your Best Friend today."

"Louise, it's good to have a friend like you. I want you to know I'm here for you!"

[To other staff members] *"Let's review resident Life Stories today. Who can tell me more about George?"*

[To another staff member] *"Anne Marie, you are full of great Knack today. I love the way you took time to smile, offer a hug, and invite that resident to join you in the garden."*

You can also add Best Friends language into key program elements. Consider reworking job descriptions to call key people "Best Friends" (see the "Memory Care Program Job Description" at the end of this chapter) or create friendship bulletin boards and posters to visually convey the importance of relationship-based care.

Dina Newsom, Expressions™ Product Manager for Prestige Care in Vancouver, Washington, has spoken about the importance of positive language throughout her long career in assisted living and memory care. For Dina, moving away from old terminology and embracing language that is respectful and affirming sets the stage for quality relationships and great programming.

> Are we working in a unit or a neighborhood? Is it a facility or community? Best Friends understand that our language has power and impacts attitudes and approaches. I would want to live in a setting with feelings of home and some warm and fuzzy, friendly and respectful language.

As we recast our culture, why don't we also consider replacing some common phrases and words still used every day in long-term care with alternatives that convey a more caring view?

- A *problem* can become a *challenge* or even an *opportunity* (reinforces that we can find solutions with creativity, as we have recommended in Chapter 7).

- A *hydration hour* can become a *Happy Hour* or *tea party* (moves it from a medical to social perspective).

- The phrase *family burden* can become *family journey* (creates more hope and optimism).

- *Respite* programs can become *respite and enrichment* programs (stressing that the family and person all benefit).
- People labeled as *feeders* (terrible!) can become *people who need dining assistance* (respectful!).
- A *patient* becomes a *person* (unless you are specifically referring to his or her time under medical care).
- A *unit* or *pod* can become a *neighborhood* (creates a community).
- A *room* can become an *apartment* (more homelike).
- A *wanderer* can become someone who is *walking with purpose* (even if we need to address their *purpose* to leave a secure place).
- *Bibs* can become *dining scarves* (keep it adult).
- *Activities* can become *moments of engagement*.
- An *in-service* can become a *class* or *learning circle* (more inclusive).
- *Problem behaviors* can become *responsive behaviors* (language that challenges us to look for root causes).

Simple changes with profound effects, don't you think?

Take Staff Training to a Higher Level

Sometimes it seems that training in the broad long-term care industry feels way behind the times. Staff managing the challenges of dementia care may receive just a few hours of training and minimal ongoing support. What training does happen may consist of little more than watching a video, hearing a short lecture, or dozing through a boring PowerPoint presentation. The emerging trend of online learning is promising when coupled with plenty of follow up, reinforcement, and evaluation.

In any dementia care program, staff should be taught the basics about dementia so they have a solid understanding of the disease. Suitable dementia training not only helps staff build skills but also develops empathy. As you strive to improve your training, consider a few of these tips adapted from the book *The Best Friends Staff*:

- *Keep it simple:* Sometimes we jam so much into one in-service that staff become overwhelmed. Focus on a few key concepts in each in-service. For example, a program on communication could discuss the importance of slowing down and speaking up, using positive body language, giving compliments, and offering simple choices. A class on Life Story could invite team members to write a short version of their own Life Story to share with the group. This type of activity helps reinforce the power of the Life Story to bring us closer together.

- *Follow up:* None of us learns very well when exposed to information just once. If a training, for example, is on fall prevention, build in some activities throughout the month to remind your staff about key principles. Establish the day after the formal training as "Fall Prevention Day" to look for trip hazards or other problems.

    Do the same for Best Friends training. If you have a training on communication skills, follow up with conversation starter cards, individual assignments, or a "Compliments Day." No matter what the topic, come up with ways to creatively reinforce lessons learned!

- *Create learning circles or classes:* Work as a team to devise some 5-minute classes on a variety of topics suitable for a stand-up meeting, perhaps a simple role-play on giving compliments or offering choices, a short discussion of Knack, or reading aloud and then discussing what Rebecca Riley used to say: "I dislike friends, family, and social workers who do not treat me as a real person." (Revisit Rebecca's Life Story in Chapter 1.)

- *Make it fun:* Programming consultant Kathy Laurenhue strives to make training fun and engaging. "I use word games, puns, even cartoon-like graphics on my handouts to keep people intrigued. Partnering staff up or breaking into small groups helps. I have not succeeded unless behavior on the job changes; relaxed and emotionally engaged class members learn more."

Knack, Lack, and Wack

Best Friends Master Trainers at Plaza Assisted Living in Honolulu, Hawaii, have a clever way to teach staff about the Knack. First, they create three handheld signs: one that says *Knack!*, one that says *Lack!*, and one that says *Wack!* (slang for something being "lame" or off course). During a training, they give each staff member a set of these signs. When the leader describes a scenario or organizes a role-play similar to the ones you read about in Chapter 5, each staff member raises a sign to vote on whether the idea is:

KNACK! (a great example of Best Friends in action)

LACK! (close, but not quite perfect)

WACK! (an example of what *not* to do in memory care!)

Sell the Benefits

Continually remind the staff around you of the benefits of the Best Friends program. Stakeholders include the administrator and corporate staff (if any), supervisors, care staff, families, and even each person with dementia.

The benefits are many. Being a Best Friend:

- encourages meaningful relationships that can touch the spirit of staff and residents
- helps make personal care more successful
- is good for the bottom line because a happier, more successful staff experiences lower turnover, and a high-quality program attracts more "customers," thus improving census
- adds to everyone's job satisfaction

One way to sell the benefits of the program to management and customers is to ask staff for testimonials that you can film with a cell phone or video recorder. For example, if a new CNA in skilled nursing or a new in-home worker hears a peer talk about how the Best Friends program is meaningful and fun, the odds are he or she will be more open to learning about the program.

It can also be powerful to remind your supervisor that an excellent program becomes a program all leaders and staff can become proud of. It's possible to go from a workplace to a caring community.

Address Barriers and Objections

Barriers exist that may slow down or stop the development of a Best Friends program. For example, a below-par housekeeping or food service program creates frustration and poor morale. Leaders may not free up adequate financial resources. Whenever possible, work with your team to address these barriers before you begin a Best Friends initiative.

We recall one community that was struggling to cover the basics. The commercial dishwasher had been broken for weeks, causing the staff to spend hours doing dishes (note that they tried to involve residents in helping, but the chore took away from other more enjoyable activities). The small back garden was full of weeds and needed mulch, taking away much of the joy of being outside. Staff requests for help seemed to be going nowhere. Remembering the old saying that a picture paints a thousand words, David Troxel suggested that the frustrated executive director take pictures of the stacked dishes and problem garden space and send them to the regional director. "Seeing those pictures, bringing those issues to life, propelled the regional director into action. The new dishwasher and mulch arrived shortly."

Other barriers are more individual in nature. Some staff—direct care staff as well as clinical staff—simply aren't ready to embrace change. The Best Friends journey will attract many supporters, but be prepared to address the objections of the one or two people ready to tell you why the program won't work.

"We Don't Have the Money"

The Best Friends approach doesn't need fancy furniture or an expensive architect. Best practices don't need to be expensive. For example, a simple walk or a side-by-side visit in the garden with a Best Friend can be an opportunity for engagement. You can create a meaningful bulletin board with old sayings on friendship, or make simple cards highlighting Life Story facts that everyone can use in everyday interactions with residents. Managers can conduct role-plays demonstrating relationship-based care (e.g., the importance of body language such as smiles and welcomed hugs) or develop some easy-to-implement training themes around the Dementia Bill of Rights. Money doesn't have to be a barrier.

"We Don't Have the Time"

Some people believe that staff whose attention is already stretched thin can't possibly implement a person-centered strategy that, in essence, asks them to slow down. Our reply is: *It only takes 30 seconds to be a little less task oriented and a little more person centered.* No matter what you are doing, it's always possible to slow down a bit and focus on the person and the experience he or she is having. Slowing down will help everything go better and may even make things go faster! Impatiently tapping your foot and pushing someone through an unpleasant routine will create resistance; the task will actually take more time.

If your job is to help someone with personal care, take some time to offer a friendly greeting, talk about a favorite subject, and show the person that you care. This almost always creates a better dynamic. With greater cooperation, you'll actually save time, and both of you will have a more rewarding experience.

"We Don't Have the Staff"

We admit it: we are idealists. In our perfect world, every program would have a one-to-one staffing ratio, team members would be highly paid, and benefits would be generous. However, even employers who affirm, recognize, and reward staff eventually discover that finding and keeping excellent staff can be hard.

When you are facing a staff shortage, it's even more important to have a good program. A few ideas:

• Use both volumes of the *The Best Friends Book of Alzheimer's Activities* to find small group activities and activities that can be done without much preparation. For example, you can set up a collage project that can be enjoyed throughout the week for one-on-one work or group work.

• Create a Top Five or Top Ten Life Story list like the one in Chapter 3 (Figure 3.3) for each resident, so that staff can at least know the basics. As we've emphasized through this book, sometimes even knowing just a few pieces of information about a person can evoke happiness and turn a *no* into a *yes*.

• You should never replace staff with volunteers, but volunteers can amplify what you do. Build your own volunteer program, matching residents to Best Friends and recruiting volunteers with similar interests to help out in your care setting. Review Chapter 9 for tips on building your volunteer program.

Turning a difficult staffing situation around can be an uphill battle. But if your work environment stresses optimism, relationships, and fun (along with good training and support), you can become an employer of choice in your marketplace.

"The Surveyors Won't Like It!"

From time to time we hear program administrators fret that the ideas contained in the Best Friends philosophy will not be in accord with state requirements ("Does a Life Story form comply with HIPAA?" "Straying from the calendar to do unstructured activities might cause us to be written up.").

There is little we (or anyone) can do if you are visited by a rogue surveyor, but a principle adopted by Virginia and David has served them well over the many years of developing and implementing programs: If your program or idea is good for the person, if it supports a rich and healthy life, it's rarely if ever "against regs."

Although David has seen situations that are frustrating, he'd rather go down fighting at times for his best ideas than not create an innovative, life-enriching program. Citations can be appealed. And if you lose one now and then, your team and families will rally behind you for doing the right thing and being an advocate for people with dementia.

"But I'm Not in Charge!"

Even if you are the only one in your community who glimpses the potential of the Best Friends approach, even if you have no support from any level of management or any other staff, in fact even if management is actively hostile toward any kind of change, you can still live out the Best Friends approach in your relationships. As your life changes, so will the lives around you.

Start by being a Best Friend to someone with dementia. Pick one or two special residents and learn their Life Stories. If you play piano, take a few minutes to play for residents in assisted living. Take someone who is in skilled nursing outside for 10 minutes to enjoy a lovely day, or turn off the television and engage a resident in conversation. The relationship will change. You'll change. So will the other person. Good things will happen because of it.

Little by little, your actions are sure to be noticed. When someone comments on why Mrs. Smith doesn't resist her shower when you are helping, you have a perfect opportunity to explain what you are doing that is getting different results. And you can refer the questioner to this book or the Best Friends approach website (www.bestfriends approach.com), or offer a copy of the Dementia Bill of Rights. Ideally your individual modeling and championship will begin to turn the tide, but if not, you can at least feel very good that you are bringing your Knack and your values to the program and that your actions are fostering happiness in others.

Celebrate Your Successes

Be sure to celebrate successes as you move through your culture change calendar. Sing or listen to popular songs about friendship (James Taylor's rendition of "You've Got a Friend," Alan Gold's "Thank You for Being My Friend," or Bette Midler's inspiring version of "Wind Beneath My Wings").

Purchase greeting cards relating to friendship or create your own using famous quotes about friendship you can find on the Internet. Give them to staff members who have excelled or finished their training.

Some Best Friends adopters, including a statewide initiative in Oregon, have produced buttons that say "I Have the Knack" or "Ask me about Knack" to hand out to enthusiastic staff.

Another great way to gain visibility is to post activities from your Best Friends efforts on social media (make sure you have appropriate photo releases and permissions to post the images or names of staff members or residents). Many of us enjoy seeing our friends and families on Facebook and other social media. Your Best Friends program will get plenty of "likes."

Sustaining Your Best Friends Program

Your program is up and running. You are celebrating your successes. Suddenly, two key staff members give notice. A new regional person comes in who doesn't know much about the Best Friends program. What now? Even a strong program can begin to lose focus over time or begin to flounder without being "watered and fed."

Experience has taught us that sustaining a Best Friends program means practicing the principles introduced in this book—and continuing to use the same tools introduced in this chapter. Most of the recommendations for creating a Best Friends culture initiative can be repurposed to support long-term success. For example, investing in new and improved training programs can have impact over several years. The work in creating and maintaining Life Stories will pay dividends for many years. Updating your first 12-month plan by developing new annual plans with new and improved goals will help you continue progressing.

We've shared a few more ideas in "21 Ways to Sustain a Best Friends Program." These Best Friends principles and practices will nurture your long-term success. So will the perspectives of colleagues in the next section, who share ways in which they keep their programs vibrant and effective.

Keep the Focus

Set up a standing work group or Best Friends committee that meets monthly. Besides ensuring an ongoing focus on Best Friends culture, it can be an asset when concerns are raised or resources are needed. A recommendation from the work group (e.g., we need to buy some

How Elmcroft Senior Living Created and Sustains Its Best Friends Program

Gerry Jackson, director of training at Elmcroft Senior Living, is a true champion of the Best Friends approach. Gerry led Elmcroft in the process of integrating the approach into its Heartland Village memory care neighborhoods. Supporting the importance of Life Story, Gerry is committed to "helping every resident's present be as meaningful as their past."

Gerry calls the Best Friends approach "our sole philosophy on care delivery in our Heartland Village memory care program." To create and sustain its Best Friends program, Elmcroft:

- Identified a core group of people who not only embraced key elements of Best Friends but also stood among their peers as leaders for memory support care provision. "We jokingly called them 'sneezers,' as their spreading the word about the use of all components of the Best Friends approach infected everyone."

- Arranged for the core group to be trained in the Best Friends approach at the annual Best Friends™ Approach Institute for Master Trainer Certification.

- Used the Master Trainers to begin training throughout their company.

- After the initial trainings, developed a full and thoughtful implementation timeline for the Best Friends approach, setting specific goals related to training, activities, and the overall program.

- Trained all regional directors of operations and quality service managers as Best Friends Master Trainers. This ensured that managers understood the program goals and could provide appropriate mentoring, modeling, and coaching throughout the company. This also supported accountability, helping everyone achieve a common vision and serve a common purpose.

- Trains each new associate through in-person training and video testimonies from care partners, staff, and family members who have witnessed the key elements of Best Friends in action, thereby helping new staff understand and master the key Best Friends principles.

new music resources) often carries more weight than a recommendation from a single person.

Many companies sponsor an annual dementia care program retreat with guest speakers and team-building activities. Incorporating planning, work groups, and retreats into your annual budget and calendar provides a focal point for your program each year.

Old Idea vs. New Idea Programs

Are you working in an Old Idea Program? Use this list, even if it's a bit painful, to think about your current situation and begin to create your vision for a Best Friends program. Don't be discouraged if many of your answers are on the left side of this list. We all have to begin somewhere. If you use many of the ideas in this chapter, you will find your program evolving into one that exemplifies many contemporary ideas of quality dementia care. You will also find yourself enjoying your work more.

Old Idea Program	New Idea Program/Best Friends Way
Hires warm bodies/anyone	Innovative recruitment
Little or no training	Investment in training
Minimal wages	Competitive wages
Only activity staff do activities	Everyone does activities, brings in their own interests and skills
Training by lecture and video only	Interactive, innovative training
Little or no follow-through	Knowledge is reinforced by modeling, practicums, small group work, or other methods
No feedback from staff	Training evaluated
Quick entry into job	Orientation about program history, philosophy, and mission; start right out with skill building
Task oriented	Person oriented
Staff only do assigned tasks	Self-starters, take initiative, team-oriented
Staff struggle in interactions with residents	Staff experience successes
Staff feel put upon, under siege	Staff feel appreciated
High turnover	Good staff stay
Low morale	High morale
Resists change	New ideas welcome
Shame-based management	Reward-based management
"Looking for mistakes"	"Looking for successes"
Many resident behaviors reflect distress, anxiety, restlessness	Residents seem happy, enjoying and feeling secure in the community

Train, Coach, and Train Some More

Mark Steele, president and CEO of Salemtowne Retirement Community in Winston-Salem, North Carolina, suggests that a key to sustaining good programs is building leaders at all levels in the organization: "Providing training and coaching about leadership to your key team members helps them be better communicators and model and mentor excellence. It also helps fulfill many staff members' ideals to make their community a better place for all—a caring community."

One way he helps staff learn new concepts and discuss and share ways to put them into practice is through an employee book club: "I choose some of my favorite books relating to leadership, get copies for my leadership team, we read the book, and then have regular discussions about key chapters or concepts."

When Dan Kuhn worked for the Greater Illinois Chapter of the Alzheimer's Association, he helped develop and introduce "Comfort Care for Advanced Dementia," an outstanding education program relating to end-of-life care for people with dementia. During the rollout, he noticed that the most effective partner organizations had progressive and talented leaders who were fully invested in the program and who were, according to Dan, "not just top down, but collegial and inclusive. My key piece of advice is, getting leadership on board is essential."

Courtney Way, RN, training and development manager for Heritage Community of Kalamazoo, has been a longtime advocate:

> It may seem overwhelming when you first attempt to introduce Best Friends to your community, but I encourage you to step back and look at the "big picture." When you realize every member of your team touches the lives of residents, the effort is worth it. Heritage has trained security guards, housekeepers, servers, and many nontraditional individuals, encouraging them to be Best Friends champions. The response to this approach, through comments and letters from friends and their families, has been amazing.

Make Resources Available

Tom Alaimo, vice president of memory care operations (Life Guidance®) for Atria Senior Living, believes that part of sustainability is to provide staff easy access to information, resources, and training:

> We purchased hundreds of copies of the Best Friends activity books for our communities to utilize, and over time these books were offered to families and others in

Create a Best Friends "Job Description"

We encourage you to add language about the Best Friends approach to your job descriptions. Here's how ABHOW describe the care partners who work in their memory support program, The Grove.

Memory Support Program "Best Friend"

General Statement of Job

Under general supervision, provides direct resident care and assists in residents' activities of daily living and scheduled Memory Support Program activities as a "Best Friend." Develops awareness of residents' interests and needs and assists residents to maximize their independence and participation. Actively incorporates "The Best Friends Model" and The Grove Philosophy for Memory Support . . . into the daily rhythm of life of residents with dementia. Duties and assignments may be adjusted at the discretion of the Memory Support Director and/or The Grove Program Coordinator.

Reports to: Memory Support Program "Best Friend Team Leader"

Essential functions: The following duties are normal for this position. These are not to be construed as exclusive or all-inclusive. Other duties may be required and assigned.

- Engages in the "treatment" philosophy of The Grove, as described in *The Best Friends Approach to Dementia Care*, defined as loving care, involvement in activity programming, and one-on-one engagement; establishing relationships; knowing and using resident Life Stories; effective communication; and a positive, can-do attitude toward behavior that is challenging.

- Participates with residents as they complete specific tasks related to personal hygiene, bathing, and dressing; assists in ambulating, grooming, helping with activities, and responding to emotional needs.

- Actively engages residents in participation in daily activities that are part of resident's rhythm of daily life.

an effort to benefit our seniors with memory impairments. Today, while we still purchase some copies, we utilized technology and partnered with the publisher to offer every Atria community virtual access to the Best Friends activity books through our internal Intranet. Additionally, we offer our teams a virtual eLearning platform with training videos that reinforce the Best Friends approach to dementia care. In turn, this helped our community leaders develop great programming for our residents, effective training for our staff, and a true Best Friends environment for our residents.

Tom has also found other solutions in technology, using online surveys such as SurveyMonkey® to gain ongoing input and buy-in and filming short videos about Best Friends for the company Intranet. "This has improved access to our key programming and training materials so everyone can help us build a true Best Friends environment," he says.

Bringing It All Together: Americare

Americare, an early champion of the Best Friends philosophy, owns senior living communities (from independent living to skilled nursing) in Kansas, Missouri, Tennessee, Illinois, and Mississippi. Their memory care assisted living communities are called The Arbors.

Tina Buckley, divisional nurse consultant, says that the Best Friends approach supports Americare's goal to create hometown experiences: "We want our residents to experience an environment that evokes family and the hospitality of a friendly hometown. That's why Best Friends and its focus on relationships is an ideal care delivery and training model for our memory care communities."

Early on, Americare's management recognized that launching a program can be the easy part; sustaining a program is the challenge. Jean Summers, senior vice president for the assisted living division, outlines some of the company's strategies for accountability and sustainability:

- *Training:* Americare arranges for key leaders to become trained and certified as Best Friends Master Trainers. In turn, these leaders bring their expertise to their local communities, offering 18 hours of training on the Best Friends philosophy for each new team member in the first 90 days of employment. Jean notes, "We really wanted to do something above and beyond. The result is that our care partners approach their day with more confidence and skill."

- *Best Friends Pledge:* Staff are asked to sign a pledge that they will practice the Best Friends approach, support the Best Friends™ Dementia Bill of Rights, and contribute meaningfully to a hometown environment. Jean says, "We want to stress to our team members the importance of putting the 'person before the task.'"

- *The Artifacts: The Americare Artifacts of Best Friends Approach* is a tool, created by a large work group, that supports and evaluates the quality of all aspects of its dementia care program. "It's our company document that outlines what we want to see when Best Friends is

21 Ways to Sustain a Best Friends Program

1. Create a mentoring program to help new employees better understand Best Friends.

2. Encourage your team to "like" the Best Friends approach on Facebook to see ongoing news and stories about Best Friends and high-quality dementia care.

3. Design a Best Friends bulletin board to give monthly updates and share success stories.

4. Publish a Best Friends newsletter for your families and staff.

5. Develop a Best Friends volunteer program encouraging friendly visiting or other support for people with dementia.

6. Hold occasional contests to encourage friendly competition (e.g., have each building submit a collage on friendship and vote on the best).

7. Once a quarter, update all Life Stories.

8. Profile the Life Story of a person in your program each month (and a staff member, too).

9. Sponsor a monthly family night in order to share news and program updates.

10. Hold an annual retreat to build teams and spread best practices.

11. Collect and share old sayings about friendship (widely available on the Internet or at the greeting card section in your grocery store).

12. Develop Best Friends badges or pins for employees who have achieved certain goals or finished your internal training.

13. Change your job descriptions to add Best Friends language (e.g., stressing that it's everyone's job to engage the people with dementia you serve).

14. Share with your families copies of the family care partner edition of this book: *A Dignified Life: The Best Friends Approach to Alzheimer's Care.*

15. Create a poster of the Best Friends™ Dementia Bill of Rights and develop training exercises and programs to teach staff about its importance (or have everyone sign the poster to show their commitment to its principles).

16. Choose key staff members to attend the annual Best Friends™ Approach Institute for Master Trainer Certification.

17. Have some fun teaching the concept of Knack, printing up "I have the Knack" buttons or debating Knack vs. No-Knack scenarios.

Continued

18. Invite your employees to create short video clips using their cell phones to describe how they've been Best Friends to a person in the past year. Share these online and in team trainings.

19. Each month, pick activities to do from *The Best Friends Book of Alzheimer's Activities* to help staff get into the Best Friends spirit and philosophy.

20. Read and share the brief stories along the page margins in *The Best Friends Staff* that describe successes from around the world in using the approach.

21. Write an annual report demonstrating your program's impact on your workplace culture, programming, family satisfaction, and business success.

in place," Jean says. "The evaluation tool, completed twice a year, allows us to track our success and identify any areas that need attention."

Tina and Jean shared the following stories of how the Best Friends approach has influenced care in two senior living communities:

The Arbors at Victorian Place of Washington, in Washington, Missouri, had a resident who could be disruptive to the ongoing daily programs. Life Story work revealed that the resident had learned to play the harmonica at a young age and even played it in Sunday school. Staff started to make sure she had the harmonica in her pocket. When staff could see her anxiety rising, they asked her to play a song. This calmed her and also pleased other residents and staff. A few tunes a day stopped almost all of the behavior that was challenging for the community.

At The Arbors at Bluff Creek Terrace in Columbia, Missouri, there was a resident who had to be taken to the emergency room. "She was frightened and out of her normal routine," Tina says. "Her behavior was so concerning to the hospital that the medical team placed her in the behavioral unit." Americare staff came to the hospital and dropped off a number of her favorite things as well as her Life Story information. Using these, the hospital team was able to turn around the various behaviors and help their patient feel safe and supported.

Tina notes that Americare now provides in-services to the hospital team, "and we've learned to always send out Life Story information with our residents when they have to be hospitalized."

Americare has found the Best Friends philosophy a real point of difference for market success, but even more important, a great tool for achieving culture change. "Ultimately, Best Friends benefits our residents, staff, and families," Jean says.

Conclusion

The Best Friends approach is a culture, a system of values that can transform an environment and all of the relationships within it. It's a way of living and relating that can make life better for everybody—staff, people with dementia, care partners, and families.

David Troxel recalls consulting for a program in which just about everything was going wrong. The executive director was floundering. The wrong nurse headed the nursing department. Teams were deeply dysfunctional. Direct care staff who desperately wanted to learn the Best Friends approach were not supported by their superiors. They expressed disappointment in the lack of supplies, inadequate training, and bosses who they labeled as uncaring.

In the middle of these problems, one CNA began to bring her favorite music to the program and created a weekly dance group. Other staff created Top Ten Life Story cards and used them to encourage reminiscence and better communication. And the team started up a regular happy hour with a focus on the guys. Within a few weeks you could feel the difference.

Small steps can lead to big changes, as Virginia Bell discovered many years ago after being told by everyone that a day center for people with dementia would never work. Proof positive that a Best Friends culture can be nurtured for decades is that the Best Friends™ Day Center is now more than 30 years old. As participants and volunteers have come and gone, Virginia and the talented staff and volunteers of the Best Friends team have sustained the program by focusing on, and always practicing, the basics.

At every step of the way, everyone involved in the center has perceived their work as meaningful. Your program can flourish, too, when everyone sees their work as something that not only earns a living, but also feeds the spirit. That is the best part of Best Friends: it helps us find success and enjoy our work lives more. When those two ingredients are in place, your program will survive and prosper for many years.

CHAPTER 11

Conclusion

David Troxel once witnessed a powerful interchange between a resident and a CNA care partner working in a memory support community in Atlanta, Georgia. "You look so pretty today in your pink sweater," the CNA said. Expressing surprise and holding her hands to her chest, the resident replied, "You've made my day!" A moment later the resident added, "I just want to say to you that you are *wonderful*." The staff member smiled and said, "Now *you* have made my day!" In the break room, the staff member told David, "I have a husband, two kids, and a brother and sister. Nobody at *home* tells me I am wonderful." The CNA discovered the amazing result of living out the Best Friends™ approach. One moment you are the Best Friend to someone with dementia, and the next moment that person is a Best Friend to you!

Informed Love

Celebrating the 30th anniversary of the Best Friends™ Day Center in 2014 prompted us to reflect on the joys of working in the often tough and challenging arena of dementia care. For us, joy comes from the dedicated and compassionate people we meet, like Dr. Nori Graham, the well-regarded English physician and distinguished past president of Alzheimer's Disease International. At the center's 30th anniversary gala, Dr. Graham praised the Best Friends approach and added her own take on it by saying that outstanding dementia care really just comes down to "informed love."

203

We interpret "informed love" to mean that care partners with Knack learn all they can about dementia care and apply that knowledge to forge authentic relationships with a person with dementia. Throughout this second edition of *The Best Friends Approach to Dementia Care*, we have showcased how we as care partners can be Best Friends to persons with dementia. Now we'd like to highlight the unexpected benefit of practicing the Best Friends approach—gaining a Best Friend in return.

> Elna, a retired anthropologist who was an early participant in the Best Friends™ Day Center, was paired with James, a student volunteer. James no longer went to regular high school but attended an alternative continuation program. He and some of the other young volunteers from his school looked pretty tough. Many had had trouble with the law. At first we wondered what kind of Best Friends young James and his cohort would make. Would they show up on time? Would their rough edges ruffle a few feathers? What on Earth would they talk about, across the span of three generations? Would our day center participants with dementia feel uncomfortable?
>
> Eventually we realized that our own filters and prejudices were making *us* uncomfortable. Although we, and some of our staff and volunteers, were a bit uptight, our participants with dementia didn't care a whit about tattoos, scruffy beards, or eccentric haircuts and clothes. They just saw the young people as young people, and Elna gave James unconditional love.
>
> James thrived in the program. With Elna's attention and support, he became a very successful student volunteer. As his program wound down, he told us something startling: being part of the Best Friends program was the first success he had ever experienced in his 18 years on the planet. Being a Best Friend to Elna—and enjoying Elna's friendship—made a big difference in his life. The Best Friends approach transformed James, too!

It's no accident that our book on staffing has the subtitle *Building a Culture of Care in Alzheimer's Programs.* This is what the Best Friends approach is all about. It feeds the spirit not only of the person with dementia but also of staff and families. One friend said to us recently, "I practice the Best Friends approach primarily for me. It helps me find purpose and greater enjoyment in my job!"

Looking Ahead

Dementia care has changed significantly since the first edition of this book. How exciting to ponder what the next 20 years will bring! Perhaps there will be major advances in prevention strategies and medications—perhaps even an effective treatment or cure for one or more of the dementias. Of course, there is the sobering possibility that we may be exactly where we are now, since Alzheimer's disease and other dementias have proven very tough to conquer.

What might this future look like? We are encouraged by a global movement supported by Alzheimer's Disease International and the World Health Organization called Dementia-Friendly Communities that educates residents in towns and cities to understand dementia. As part of these initiatives, services and public awareness are expanded. Community members, such as students, shopkeepers, cab drivers, and health and safety officials, work to foster independence and safety for residents with dementia. Imagine a multigenerational place where younger people are sensitive to the needs of older adults and ready to lend a helping hand.

Is it just a dream? Yes and no. In South Korea thousands of people, including teenagers, have been trained to provide elder care and help support people with dementia. In England and Wales, more than a million people have volunteered and been trained to be Dementia Friends to support neighbors with dementia. Everywhere we go, the stigma surrounding dementia is in decline, and support and acceptance are on the upswing.

Statistics show that approximately one-third of us will ultimately develop dementia. Unless we find a breakthrough treatment, we will certainly need to look at new ideas and new models to support the millions who will be affected. From our own experience over the past 20 years, we take pride in knowing that many of the best ideas will come from person- and relationship-centered approaches such as Best Friends.

Thank You for Sharing Our Journey

We want to thank you, the reader, for taking this journey with us. It has been truly encouraging to see the Best Friends approach take off, not only in the United States but also internationally, and we are truly inspired by all of the e-mails, letters, and phone calls we receive from folks who tell us how our work has helped them make a tough journey—and come out on top.

We have so loved revisiting this first work of ours. We were surprised at how much of the foundational work is still relevant and are glad for the opportunity to update the book's contents to reflect both our development as well as developments in our field.

Yet as we conclude this book, the closing paragraphs from our first edition still ring true:

The Best Friends model was created primarily for family and professional care partners coping with the effects of Alzheimer's disease, but there are lessons in it for everyone. There is great value in being totally present for another individual. There is great value in getting the most out of every moment, every day. There is great value in good communication. There is great value in honoring an individual's Life Story. There is great value in giving care to another.

Because any of us can be touched by Alzheimer's disease, can have bad things happen to us, our friends, and our families, the ultimate message the authors wish to convey is this: We should treat everyone important to us as we would our own Best Friend.

Biographies

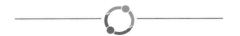

Velma Beatty (1930–)

Velma was born August 15, 1930, in Nicholasville, Kentucky. She likes to say that she was born on Kissin' Ridge. She was the only girl of four children and likes to talk about growing up with all boys. She and her "husband to be" met on a blind date, and it was love at first sight. They soon married and became parents of two children, Gary and Karen. She cherished her favorite thing: being with her husband and children. The family moved a lot during their early years, and Velma was always ready for a new adventure. During those years, she has often been quoted as saying, "Just wait and let me get my purse."

Velma often worked outside the home to supplement the family income, but she was also a social butterfly. She loves to have a good time, always enjoys music, is a good dancer, and has friends galore. Her dog, Chester, is her baby now. She's a very sweet, easygoing person; but when she digs her heels in, it's a firm I'm-not-going-to-do-it answer.

Russell Doudt (1926–2015)

Russell was born in Newark, New Jersey, where his dad was a coal miner. He went into the Air Corp before he finished high school. He spent time in the Pacific working on reconnaissance missions. After his work in the Air Corp, he finished high school and graduated from Newark College with a degree in mechanical engineering. He met his wife Marian at a dance. They married and became parents of two children, Russell Daniel and Vivian.

Russell liked to travel to Hawaii and Arizona with his wife. He liked to talk about putting his father's trains under the Christmas tree each year. He was very social, enjoyed talking about the war, loved Bluegrass

music, loved cats, and was wild about his dog, Peta. He loved seafood
and sweets even more. Russell grew up in the Catholic Church.

Robert Steele (1936–)

Robert, born in the Philippines, likes to be called Bob. His father was a
colonel in the Army. Bob grew up with his aunt Connie and his grandmother. After high school in Staunton, Virginia, he went to UCLA,
where he flunked out. His father told him either get a job or go into the
military. Bob went to the Naval Academy and served in the Navy for 20
years. He then worked as a consultant through government contracts.
Bob is married to Darlene and has two children by a previous marriage.

Bob likes anything to do with the U.S. Civil War. He is a member
of the Civil War Round Table. He enjoys researching his family tree and
loves any kind of sport. He is easygoing and loves kidding around. He
enjoyed taking many trips. His favorite trip was a 12-day cruise on the
Rhone river. Bob has been very active in the Presbyterian Church.

Ruth Eveland (1932–)

Ruth was born in 1932 in Newark, New Jersey. Her mother was a book-
keeper and her father worked for a heating and oil company. She attended Barrington High School in New Jersey, and her best friend was
Norma Hoffman. Ruth's favorite subject was English literature. Later
on, Ruth was a 3rd and 5th grade teacher. She enjoyed being with the
children. Her husband was in the Air Force, so she spent much time at
the Dover Air Force Base. They were parents of one child, Diane. Ruth's
husband is deceased. Ruth's two grandchildren, Dylan and Shannon,
are very special to her. She loves animals and has a cat named Pele. She
spent time breeding black Labrador Retrievers and Great Pyrenees.

Ruth has a pleasing disposition and likes to be included when decisions are being made. She enjoys talking about her dogs and will spend
long periods of time looking at pictures of animals and her favorite cars.
She loves to exercise, especially walking.

Stephen Troyer (1944–2015)

Stephen liked to be called Steve. He was born in Fort Wayne, Indiana. His mother was a secretary and his father owned real estate. Steve

graduated from Purdue University and loved being known as a Boiler Maker, the name of their sports team. He continued his education and received his master's from Illinois University. After graduation, Steve went to work for IBM, first in Poughkeepsie, New York, and later in Lexington, Kentucky. Steve had two daughters with his wife Carolyn. He retired from IBM in 2005.

Steve was a very intelligent person and always a very hard worker. He loved taking care of any electrical work around the house. Some of his other favorite things to do included being with family, traveling (especially to Disney World, Williamsburg, Virginia, or any beach vacation), watching sports, playing bridge, reading spy novels and about American history, woodworking, taking walks, and collecting beer cans. Steve endeared himself to his new friends at the Best Friends Day Center.

Joan Wyzenbeek (1930–2014)

Joan grew up in a low-income family and eventually dropped out of high school. However, as an adult, she earned a GED and enrolled at the University of Cincinnati. After being granted a bachelor's equivalency, Joan attended United Theological Seminary in Dayton, Ohio, and received a master's of Divinity degree. She served churches in both Ohio and Florida. She was later recruited to teach courses at Eckert College in St. Petersburg, Florida, where she became a very popular professor.

When one congregation gave Joan a toast, she said, "The reason I went into the ministry is because I didn't make it in show business." She had indeed studied acting and dance and relished any chance to appear before an audience. She loved playing a stripper in the musical Gypsy. She was often teased about how her acting role and her ministry role related to each other. She always had a witty answer. Joan was loving and thoughtful and a friend to all, especially her longtime partner, Pat Ritz.

Suggested Resources

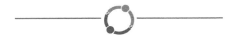

Resources on The Best Friends™ Approach

Bell, V., & Troxel, D. (2001). *The Best Friends Staff: Building a Culture of Care in Alzheimer's Programs*. Baltimore: Health Professions Press.

Bell, V., & Troxel, D. (2012). *A Dignified Life: The Best Friends Approach to Alzheimer's Care (A Guide for Care Partners)*. Deerfield Beach, FL: Health Communications, Inc.

Bell, V., Troxel, D., Cox, T., & Hamon, R. (2004). *The Best Friends Book of Alzheimer's Activities, Volume One*. Baltimore: Health Professions Press.

Bell, V., Troxel, D., Cox, T., & Hamon, R. (2007). *The Best Friends Book of Alzheimer's Activities, Volume Two*. Baltimore: Health Professions Press.

Bell, V., & Troxel, D. (2008). *Los Mejores Amigos*. The Spanish translation of *The Best Friends Approach to Alzheimer's Care* (1st edition). Mexico City, Mexico: Editorial Herder.

Greater Kentucky and Southern Indiana Alzheimer's Association. (2007). *The Best Friends DVD*. Produced by the Greater Kentucky and Southern Indiana Alzheimer's Association.

Bell, V., & Troxel, D. (2014). *The Best Friends™ Daily Planner.* Baltimore: Health Professions Press.

Best Friends Approach website: **www.bestfriendsapproach.com**

Health Professions Press Best Friends approach resource and training portal: http://bestfriends.healthpropress.com/

Best Friends on Facebook: **www.facebook.com/bestfriendsapproach**

Best Friends on Twitter: @bestfriends

Web Resources and Recommended Organizations

Alzheimer's Association (**www.alz.org**): The website of the leading Alzheimer's organization in the United States. A resource-rich and informative site for persons with dementia, families, and professionals. Resources that are particularly helpful are its publication of an annual report on the impact of dementia, online training with its CARES program, and links to local resources. Information is also available in a variety of languages, along with a 24/7 Helpline (800-272-3900).

Alzheimer's Foundation of America (AFA) (**www.alzfdn.org**): AFA unites more than 2,400 organizations supporting persons with dementia and their care partners. AFA sponsors a national memory screening day and offers helpful links to Alzheimer's societies, day centers, and care management organizations, often in more rural areas.

American Society on Aging (ASA) (**www.asaging.org**): A professional membership organization with informative publications, interest groups, online workshops, and annual conferences for professionals in the fields of aging and long-term care.

Dementia Advocacy and Support Network International (DASNI) (**www.dasninternational.org**): An Internet-based support and advocacy network for persons with dementia, including online discussion groups and forums.

Family Caregiver Alliance (**www.caregiver.org**): A well-regarded national, nonprofit organization that provides care partners with helpful information and resources. The site also offers useful information for lesbian, gay, bisexual, and transgender (LGBT) care partners.

International Council on Activity Aging (ICAA) (**www.icaa.cc**): ICAA connects a community of like-minded organizations and professionals who share the goals of changing society's perceptions of aging and improving the quality of life for aging baby boomers and older adults within seven dimensions of wellness (emotional, vocational, physical, spiritual, intellectual, social, environmental). The council supports professionals with education, information, resources, and tools so that they can achieve optimal success.

National Council of Certified Dementia Care Practitioners (NCCDP) (**www.nccdp.org**): A provider of education and training for professionals in the field of dementia.

Pioneer Network (**www.pioneernetwork.net**): The leading group providing research and advocacy on culture change in long-term care. Offers excellent workshops as well as an annual conference. The website also shares research on the benefits of and financial case for culture change.

Services & Advocacy for GLBT Elders (SAGE) (**www.sageusa.org**): SAGE is the largest and oldest organization in the United States dedicated to improving the lives of lesbian, gay, bisexual, and transgender (LGBT) older adults. They provide excellent information and training programs for organizations.

Alzheimer's Disease International (**www.alz.co.uk**): The leading organization representing Alzheimer's societies from around the world. Good information about the global impact of dementia, along with links to societies and best practices from around the world, including Canada, Mexico, and Great Britain.

Alzheimer Society Canada (**www.alzheimer.ca**): The leading education, support, and advocacy group in Canada. They offer resources in English and French.

Alzheimer's Association of Australia (**www.fightdementia.org.au**): Publishers of the helpful "Dementia Language Guidelines," which includes suggestions for "accurate, respectful, inclusive, empowering and non-stigmatizing" language to use when discussing dementia. Download the guidelines at **https://fightdementia.org.au/sites/default/files/full-language-guidelines.pdf**

Activity and Programming Resources

Activity Connection (**www.activityconnection.com**): An online resource for recreational therapists and activities professionals. They offer creative and engaging activities along with current materials on brain health and fitness.

Alzheimer's Resource Center of Connecticut (**www.alzheimersresourcecenter.org**): Producers of the DVD *Dining with Friends,*" which can help you create a lovely, social, and respectful dining experience for persons with dementia.

Alzheimer's Store (**www.alzstore.com**): Innovative products and supplies for family and professional care partners that are good for in-home, day, and residential settings.

Eldercare Conversations (**www.eldercareconversations.com**): Downloadable audio interviews on a variety of topics, including activities and volunteerism.

Meet Me at MoMA (Museum of Modern Art in New York) (**www.moma.org/meetme**): A groundbreaking program that encourages persons with dementia to visit museums. MoMA's program can inspire local efforts to add art to your programming.

Music and Memory (**www.musicandmemory.org**): Inspired by the documentary *Alive Inside*, this organization promotes the evidence-based benefits of music for persons with dementia.

Wiser Now (**www.wisernow.com**): Offers training and programming resources, product reviews, and stimulating games and exercises. A core product is MindPlay Connections, with more than 75 downloadable, printable titles. Wiser Now is also the creator of the *Creative Mind Play Collections*, featuring three separate CD-ROM collections containing 130 printable activities and exercises (available at www .healthpropress.com/cmp).

Recommended Readings

Avadian, B. (2005). *Where's my shoes? My father's walk through Alzheimer's*. Lancaster, CA: North Star Books.

Barrick, A., Rader, J., Hoffer, D., Sloane, P., & Biddle, S. (2008). *Bathing without a battle: Person-directed care of individuals with dementia, 2nd ed.* New York: Springer Publishing Company.

Brawley, E. (2005). *Design innovations for aging and Alzheimer's*. New York: Wiley.

Carpenter, M. (2012). *Confidence to Care*. Omaha, NB: Home Instead Publishing.

Brackey, J. (2008). *Creating moments of joy for the person with Alzheimer's or dementia: A journal for caregivers, 4th ed.* West Lafayette, IN: Purdue University Press.

Bryden, C. (2005). *Dancing with dementia*. London: Jessica Kingsley Publishers.

de Geest, G. (2007). *The living dementia case-study approach: Caregivers discover what works and what doesn't*. Vancouver: Trafford Publishing.

Fazio, S. (2008). *The enduring self in people with Alzheimer's: Getting to the heart of individualized care*. Baltimore: Health Professions Press.

Huebner, B. (Ed.) (2012). *I remember better when I paint: Art and Alzheimer's (Opening Doors, Making Connections)*. Glen Echo, MD: Bethesda Communications Group and New Publishing Partners.

Killick, E., & Sellick, J. (2011). *Creativity and communication in persons with dementia: A practical guide*. London: Jessica Kingsley Publishers.

Kitwood, T. (1997). *Dementia reconsidered*. Birmingham, UK: Open University Press.

Kriseman, N. (2014). *The mindful caregiver: Finding ease in the caregiving journey*. Lanham, MD: Rowman & Littlefield.

Kuhn, D. (2013). *Alzheimer's early stages: First steps for family, friends, and caregivers, 3rd ed.* Alameda, CA: Hunter House.

Larsen, B. (2006). *Movement with meaning: A multi-sensory approach for individuals with early-stage Alzheimer's disease*. Baltimore: Health Professions Press.

Levine Madori, L. (2012). *Transcending Dementia Through the TTAP Method*. Baltimore: Health Professions Press.

Laurenhue, K. (2007). *Getting to know the life stories of older adults. Activities for building relationships*. Baltimore: Health Professions Press.

Lustbader, W. (2011). *Life gets better: The unexpected pleasure of growing older*. New York: Penguin Group.

Mast, B. (2011). *Whole person dementia assessment*. Baltimore: Health Professions Press.

O'Brien, G. (2014). *On Pluto: Inside the mind of Alzheimer's*. Brewster, MA: Codfish Press.

Potts, D.C. (Ed.). (2014). *Seasons of caring: Meditations for Alzheimer's and dementia caregivers*. Chevy Chase, MD: ClergyAgainstAlzheimer's.

Power, G.A. (2017). *Dementia beyond drugs: Changing the culture of care, 2ⁿᵈ ed.* Baltimore: Health Professions Press.

Power, G.A. (2017). *Dementia beyond disease: Enhancing well-being, revised edition.* Baltimore: Health Professions Press.

Richards, M. (2011). *Caresharing: A reciprocal approach to caregiving and care receiving in the complexities of aging, illness or disability.* Woodstock, VT: Skylight Paths Publishing.

Sheehy, G. (2010). *Passages in caregiving: Turning chaos into confidence.* New York: William Morrow.

Simard, J. (2013). *The end-of-life Namaste care program for people with dementia, 2ⁿᵈ ed.* Baltimore: Health Professions Press.

Snyder, L. (2010). *Living your best with early-stage Alzheimer's: An essential guide.* Northbeach, MN: Sunrise River Press.

Snyder, L. (2009). *Speaking our minds: What it's like to have Alzheimer's.* Baltimore: Health Professions Press.

Spencer, B., & White, L. (2015). *Coping with behavior change in dementia: A family caregiver's guide.* Santa Rosa, CA: Whisp Publications.

Spencer, B., & White, L. (2006). *Moving a relative with memory loss.* Santa Rosa, CA: Whisp Publications.

Swaffer, K. (2016). *What the hell happened to my brain? Living beyond dementia.* London: Jessica Kingsley Publishers.

Taylor, R. (2006). *Alzheimer's from the inside out.* Baltimore: Health Professions Press.

Thomas, W. (2004). *What are old people for? How elders will save the world.* Acton, MA: VanderWyk and Burnham.

Zeisel, J. (2010). *I'm still here: A new philosophy of Alzheimer's care.* New York: Avery.

Zgola, J. (2001). *Bon appetite: The joy of dining.* Baltimore: Health Professions Press.

Index

Note: *b* indicates boxes, *f* figures, *p* photos, *t* tables.